tterhouse
1/21/10
$45.95

W9-CDC-304

INTERACTIVE CASE STUDIES IN

Health
Communication

WITHDRAWN

Michael P. Pagano PA-C, PhD
Assistant Professor

Department of Communication
Fairfield University
Fairfield, Connecticut

CUMBERLAND COUNTY COLLEGE LIBRARY
PO BOX 1500
VINELAND, NJ 08362-1500

JONES AND BARTLETT PUBLISHERS
Sudbury, Massachusetts
BOSTON   TORONTO   LONDON   SINGAPORE

R
118
P343
2009

World Headquarters

Jones and Bartlett Publishers
40 Tall Pine Drive
Sudbury, MA 01776
978-443-5000
info@jbpub.com
www.jbpub.com

Jones and Bartlett Publishers
Canada
6339 Ormindale Way
Mississauga, Ontario L5V 1J2
Canada

Jones and Bartlett Publishers
International
Barb House, Barb Mews
London W6 7PA
United Kingdom

Jones and Bartlett's books and products are available through most bookstores and online booksellers. To contact Jones and Bartlett Publishers directly, call 800-832-0034, fax 978-443-8000, or visit our website www.jbpub.com.

Substantial discounts on bulk quantities of Jones and Bartlett's publications are available to corporations, professional associations, and other qualified organizations. For details and specific discount information, contact the special sales department at Jones and Bartlett via the above contact information or send an email to specialsales@jbpub.com.

Copyright © 2010 by Jones and Bartlett Publishers, LLC

All rights reserved. No part of the material protected by this copyright may be reproduced or utilized in any form, electronic or mechanical, including photocopying, recording, or by any information storage and retrieval system, without written permission from the copyright owner.

The authors, editor, and publisher have made every effort to provide accurate information. However, they are not responsible for errors, omissions, or for any outcomes related to the use of the contents of this book and take no responsibility for the use of the products and procedures described. Treatments and side effects described in this book may not be applicable to all people; likewise, some people may require a dose or experience a side effect that is not described herein. Drugs and medical devices are discussed that may have limited availability controlled by the Food and Drug Administration (FDA) for use only in a research study or clinical trial. Research, clinical practice, and government regulations often change the accepted standard in this field. When consideration is being given to use of any drug in the clinical setting, the health care provider or reader is responsible for determining FDA status of the drug, reading the package insert, and reviewing prescribing information for the most up-to-date recommendations on dose, precautions, and contraindications, and determining the appropriate usage for the product. This is especially important in the case of drugs that are new or seldom used.

Production Credits

Publisher: David Cella
Acquisitions Editor: Kristine Johnson
Associate Editor: Maro Asadoorian
Production Director: Amy Rose
Senior Production Editor: Renée Sekerak
Production Assistant: Jill Morton
Senior Marketing Manager: Barb Bartoszek
Associate Marketing Manager: Lisa Gordon
Manufacturing and Inventory Control Supervisor: Amy Bacus

Composition: Arlene Apone
Cover Design: Scott Moden
Cover Images: © Orange Line Media/Dreamstime.com;
    © Kovalev Serguei/ShutterStock, Inc.;
    © Monkey Business Images/ShutterStock, Inc.;
    Background image, Robert A. Mansker/ShutterStock, Inc.
Printing and Binding: Malloy Incorporated
Cover Printing: Malloy Incorporated

Library of Congress Cataloging-in-Publication Data
Pagano, Michael P.
  Interactive case studies in health communication / by Michael P. Pagano.
      p. ; cm.
  Includes bibliographical references and index.
  ISBN 978-0-7637-6018-2
  1. Communication in medicine--Case studies. I. Title.
  [DNLM: 1. Delivery of Health Care--Case Reports. 2. Delivery of Health Care--Problems and Exercises. 3. Communication--Case Reports. 4. Communication--Problems and Exercises. 5. Health Promotion--Case Reports. 6. Health Promotion--Problems and Exercises. 7. Professional-Patient Relations--Case Reports. 8. Professional-Patient Relations--Problems and Exercises. W 18.2 P131i 2009]
  R118.P343 2009
  610.69'6--dc22
                          2008036817

6048

Printed in the United States of America
13 12 11 10 09   10 9 8 7 6 5 4 3 2 1

DEDICATION

This book is dedicated to Canera,
who taught me how to communicate with patients
and showed me how to enjoy life.

CONTENTS

PREFACE

This book is based on my 30 years of experience as a healthcare provider and my nearly 20 years of teaching health communication in medical schools, universities, and hospitals. During this time I have seen how important health communication is to healthcare providers and to health communication students. In addition, I've noticed that when health communication is discussed in classrooms, students are generally more interactive and more engaging when they work with or role play real examples of health communication.

The purpose of this text is to offer faculty, providers, and students of health communication an interactive method for exploring a wide variety of health communication interactions. The initial scenarios in each chapter are paraphrases and/or reconstructions of communication taken from observations during my three decades as a healthcare provider in hospitals, clinics, and private offices; as well as from my experiences as a patient, family member, and friend.

The goals of this interactive approach are:

1. For classes, small groups, or individuals to be able to use the examples provided here to increase awareness, contemplation, analysis, and discussion of the various topics and theories.
2. For the reader, armed with this assessment, to use critical thinking to recreate the interaction using more effective communication behaviors, and to enhance the interpersonal relationship of the interactants.
3. To develop communication strategies that seek to enhance information-sharing, trust, and goal attainment for all interactants.

Let me point out that I have heard providers often state that they have no time for more conversation with patients. Clearly, as a provider in emergency medicine and occupational medicine settings, I am acutely aware of the current time constraints placed on a wide variety of healthcare contexts. However, I have seen that with analysis, practice, and commitment, providers can enhance the information exchange that needs to occur in health communication settings and build relationships while still maintaining effective time management. In addition, just as providers can decrease the time needed for physical examinations by improving their diagnostic skills, so too can they decrease the time needed for effective communication by practicing the interpersonal and health communication behaviors needed to exchange information, empower patients, and enhance outcomes.

To aid in this effort, each chapter has a unique approach to specific communication topics or behaviors. However, all chapters include effective and ineffective examples of interpersonal communication and interpersonal relationships. Please use the Table of Contents to help you determine which topics you want to explore and practice as they apply to your reading of a traditional text or to skills that you want to enhance. I hope you will embrace the interactive aspects of this text and find them beneficial for increasing your understanding of, and your ability to assess and practice, effective health communication.

NOTE: All names used in this text are fictional.

REVIEWER RECOGNITION

Special thanks go to the reviewers of this text:

Angela Albright, PhD, RN, PMHCNS-BC
Associate Dean
College of Health and Human Services
California State University, Dominguez Hills

Maria Brann, PhD
Assistant Professor of Communication Studies
West Virginia University

A. Celeste Farr, PhD
Assistant Professor of Health Communication
North Carolina State University

Kirk Hazlett, MBA, APR
Assistant Professor of Communication
Curry College

Haywood B. Joiner, Jr., MEd, DEd, MT (ASCP)
Chair and Associate Professor
Department of Allied Health
Louisiana State University at Alexandria

Linda Kean, PhD
Associate Professor
School of Communication
East Carolina University

Mary W. Mathis, MPH
Instructor
Mercer University School of Medicine

USING THIS TEXT

This book is intended to be used as a supplement to a traditional health communication theory textbook. However, faculty and/or readers can choose to use it independently to improve analytical and critical thinking skills as well as verbal and nonverbal behaviors.

This book emphasizes the role of interpersonal communication (between two people) for exchanging information effectively and for building interpersonal relationships. It is vitally important to successful outcomes, from both a provider's and a patient's perspective, that providers develop, maintain, and enhance interpersonal relationships with patients and family members or care givers. Whether it's a one-time visit to the Emergency Department or the first visit to a pediatrician's office at the start of a nearly two-decade partnership— relationships are important to building and maintaining trust, loyalty, and collaboration.

In order to get the most out of this book, I would encourage you to use it as a truly interactive resource. Here are some suggestions:

For the classroom

- Role play the initial scenario in each chapter
- Individually analyze the communication and answer the questions that follow the interaction as fully as possible
- Discuss the class's responses in terms of communication theory, information-sharing, relationship building, and goal attainment
- Individually, or in a small group (2–3 members), create a new scenario based on class discussion
- Role play the alternate interaction from this text
- Compare the alternate version to the scenario you or your group created

- Discuss the various approaches, which aspects of each you find most effective, and why
- Discuss the questions and key points at the end of the chapter
- As a group, summarize what you discovered about the communication topic in the chapter and how health communication can be used more effectively

For a small group

- Role play the initial scenario
- Analyze the communication and answer the questions that follow the interaction as fully as possible
- Discuss the various responses in terms of communication theory, information-sharing, relationship building, and goal attainment
- Create a new scenario based on class discussion
- Role play the alternate scenario from this text
- Compare the alternate interaction to the version your group created
- Discuss the various approaches, which aspects of each you find most effective, and why
- Discuss the questions and key points at the end of the chapter
- Summarize what your group discovered about the communication topic in the chapter and how health communication can be used more effectively

Individually

- Read over the initial scenario
- Analyze the communication and answer the questions that follow the interaction as fully as possible
- Create a new scenario based on your analysis
- Read and analyze the alternate scenario from this text
- Compare the alternate interaction to the one you created
- Determine which points of each you find most important for improving the information-exchange and enhancing goal attainment for the interactants
- Respond to the questions and read the key points at the end of the chapter
- Consider what you discovered about the communication topic in the chapter and how health communication can be used more effectively

PROVIDER
COMMUNICATION

LEARNING TO TALK LIKE A HEALTHCARE PROVIDER

1

Before reading the interaction below, please consider the following topics:

Narrative
- Humans like to tell stories, especially about their health

Nonverbal communication behaviors
- Kinesics
  - Facial expressions
  - Body movements
  - Posture
  - Eye gaze
- Proxemics
  - Distance between communicators
- Artifacts
  - Clothing
  - Jewelry
  - Tattoos and piercings
  - Provider uniforms
- Paralinguistic cues
  - Tone of voice
  - Volume
  - Silence
- Haptics
  - Touch

Feedback
- Asking questions to assure understanding
- Restating what was heard for clarity
- Nonverbal behaviors to illustrate comprehension or confusion

INITIAL INTERACTION

Role play and/or analyze the following example.
Insert your name and/or profession in the appropriate blanks below.

Four students sit in chairs behind a healthcare provider, who is standing while talking to a woman seated on the end of an examination table. The female patient, Connie Jones, is clothed only in a paper gown, and staring down at her hands that are clenched together in her lap.

Provider: "Hello, Ms. Jones. I want to thank you for agreeing to let these _____ students listen to our discussion."

Ms. Jones: "No problem. I just want to feel better, and if I can help them, that's great. I just hope you can help me."

Provider: "I'm sure we can; so tell me why you're here today?"

Ms. Jones: "Well, I'm having a pain in my side and—"

Provider: "Which side?"

Ms. Jones: "It's on this side."

Provider: "When did you first notice the pain?"

Ms. Jones: "It started last week and hasn't really stopped. I was having kind of a rough week."

Provider: "How would you rate your pain? If zero were no pain and ten were the most pain you've ever had, how much would you say this pain is?"

Ms. Jones: "Uh, well, sometimes it's as high as a six, but right now it's probably more like three or four. But maybe. . ."

Provider: "Sorry, just a few more questions. Do you feel like vomiting, or have you vomited? And any diarrhea?"

Ms. Jones: "I've felt a little queasy, but I haven't thrown up. And I have diarrhea."

Provider: "So how many times a day are you having a bowel movement?"

Ms. Jones: "Two or three times, and its pretty loose."

Provider: "We call that loose stools, but not diarrhea unless it's more than five stools per day. We're almost done with the questions, but can you tell me if you've ever had any abdominal surgery?"

Ms. Jones: "No, do you think I need surgery?"

Provider: "No. When was your last period?"

Ms. Jones: "I'm pretty irregular, so I'm not sure if I had one last month or the month before."

Provider: "Are you on the pill?"

Ms. Jones: "No, but I don't think I'm pregnant."

Provider: "We'll get some blood to be sure. How about urinating—are you peeing more than usual, or burning when you pee?"

Ms. Jones: "I don't think so."

Provider:	"Well, we'll check your urine too. Any blood in your stools, or are they ever black?"
Ms. Jones:	"I haven't seen any."
Provider:	"Okay, we've got what we need. Now I'm going to have the students step out, and we'll get some blood and urine for tests, and then we'll do your examination."
Ms. Jones:	"Do you know what's wrong with me?"
Provider:	"Not yet, but I've got some ideas, and the blood and urine tests and your examination should help. Just try to relax and I'll be back in a few minutes."

Discussion Questions

1. How would you describe the communication that occurred between the provider and the patient?

   _____

   _____

   _____

2. How did the provider's interruptions of the patient's communication contribute to or detract from the provider's information gathering?

   _____

   _____

   _____

3. What did the students learn about communicating with a patient from this example?

   _____

   _____

   _____

4. Describe how the provider's nonverbal behaviors communicated his/her status and role? What specific examples support your observations?

   _____

   _____

   _____

5. What verbal communication from the patient would you like to have expanded?

   _____

   _____

   _____

6. What verbal communication from the provider would you like to change?

_____

_____

_____

7. Identify three or four behaviors (verbal and/or nonverbal) that would help to enhance an interpersonal relationship between the provider and the patient.

_____

_____

_____

8. Why is an interpersonal relationship important to provider–patient interactions?

_____

_____

_____

Interactive Activity

- Rewrite (individually or in a group) the interaction between the provider and Ms. Jones, and alter the verbal and nonverbal behaviors as needed to make the health communication exchange more effective for both participants.
- How might you improve the learning experience for the students?
- Compare your rewrite to the Alternate Interaction that follows.

Interaction Rewrite

_____

_____

_____

_____

_____

_____

_____

_____

_____

_____

ALTERNATE INTERACTION

Insert your name and/or profession in the appropriate blanks below.

The provider enters the room by himself/herself and offers to shake the patient's hand. After they shake hands, the provider sits down before speaking. The patient is seated on a chair and dressed in her clothes. The provider makes eye contact with the patient as they talk.

Provider:	"Hi, Ms. Jones. I have four _____ students who would like to observe me and listen as we talk. I'd like to know if it would be okay with you for them to come in, or if you would prefer that it just be you and me?"
Ms. Jones:	"It's fine with me. I just want to get to feeling better."
	(The provider goes outside and comes back in with four students, who sit on rolling chairs behind the provider. The provider sits down before speaking.)
Provider:	"Thanks again for agreeing to have these students listen. Now I'd like to follow-up on what you were saying before they came in. You said you wanted to get to feeling better, and that's my goal as well. So let's begin by you telling me about the reason you came in to see me today."
Ms. Jones:	"Okay, well last week I started having a pain in my right side. It started the day after I fell on the ice. I didn't notice it right away, but then when I lie down or cough—it really hurts. And my husband said I might have broken something, and I'm keeping him awake because it's hard to sleep. Sometimes the pain is so bad I get sick to my stomach. I missed work today because I just don't feel well."
Provider:	"I'm sorry you don't feel well and it sounds like it's been a really miserable few days. I heard you say that the pain is on your right side and it's worse when you're lying down or coughing. Is that right?"
Ms. Jones:	"Yes."
Provider:	"Anything else you want to tell me?"
Ms. Jones:	"No, I think that's it for now."
Provider:	"Good, now I need to ask a few questions. Then we'll examine you and get you some treatment and help you start feeling better. Have you been short of breath since this happened?"
Ms. Jones:	"A bit right after I fell, but not now."
Provider:	"Have you been coughing more than usual?"
Ms. Jones:	"No. I have allergies, so I cough every now and then, but not any more than usual."
Provider:	"Okay, any blood in your sputum?"
Ms. Jones:	"No, no blood."

Provider:	"Okay, then can you tell me about your diarrhea?"
Ms. Jones:	"It started yesterday. It's real runny and I've gone three times since yesterday, and I never go more than once a day."
Provider:	"So it's been more watery, but any sign of blood or black, tarry-looking stools?"
Ms. Jones:	"No, I'd be really scared then."
Provider:	"Well, we don't want you scared. Any pain in your stomach or abdomen?"
Ms. Jones:	"No, it's just in my side."
Provider:	"Any pain when you urinate, or any blood in your urine?"
Ms. Jones:	"No, it's just like always."
Provider:	"Okay, so let me make sure I heard everything you said. You fell on the ice last week and immediately had a pain in your right side and some shortness of breath, but the breathing got back to normal pretty fast. After that you just had pain in your side, which gets worse when you lie down or cough. You cough occasionally, but no more than you did before you fell. You haven't coughed up any blood, or had any vomiting, and you don't have any pain in your abdomen. Is that right?"
Ms. Jones:	"Yes. So what do we do now?"
Provider:	"Good question. The students and I are going to go out, and Sally will be in and get you into a gown. I'll come back and do an examination, and then I want to get a chest X-ray and see if you have any broken ribs. Does that sound okay?"
Ms. Jones:	"That sounds great. I just want to stop hurting and get some sleep."
Provider:	"Give me a little more time and we'll see what your examination and the X-ray show, but I'm confident we can reduce your pain and get you some sleep."

Follow-up Discussion

1. What elements of the alternate interaction do you think might contribute to more effective communication between the provider and patient?

_____

_____

_____

2. How does the patient's use of a narrative (her story about her fall and the pain) enhance the provider's information gathering?

_____

_____

_____

3. Is there any new information uncovered via the narrative versus the interruptions and questioning of the first example?

_____

_____

_____

4. Discuss any potential differences in the impact of the two scenarios on the students' education.

_____

_____

_____

5. What is communicated by having the patient dressed in her clothes in the alternate example?

_____

_____

_____

6. What is communicated by having the provider sit down in the second interaction?

_____

_____

_____

7. How does the provider's use of feedback, by repeating what the patient told him/her, enhance the interpersonal relationship and communication?

_____

_____

_____

8. How does the provider, in the alternate interaction, use nonverbal and verbal behaviors to enhance communication positively?

_____

_____

_____

9. How did the provider's lack of interruptions in the alternate scenario impact the communication?

_____

_____

_____

_____

Key Points

1. Training students to be able to communicate as a healthcare provider requires learning more than terminology.

2. Humans like to tell stories, and by letting patients tell their stories, providers can get more information than by interrupting with a lot of questions.

3. Nonverbal communication behaviors are critical to enhancing communication exchange and building a relationship. Making eye contact with patients, using an appropriate greeting and shaking hands, sitting rather than standing above a patient while the two converse, and having the patient clothed are all examples of nonverbal communication that encourage collaboration, minimize power imbalances, and enhance interpersonal relationship development and maintenance.

4. Using feedback to demonstrate that a provider is listening, and to assure that the message she/he heard is what the sender intended to communicate, is another important interpersonal communication behavior. Feedback is valuable for both the provider, who can assure effective communication, and for patients, because it clearly demonstrates that the provider was listening or that there was a miscommunication that needs clarification or restating.

5. Interrupting is a masculine-gendered trait, and it often limits the exchange of information rather than improves it. It also nonverbally communicates that the provider who interrupts has all the power in the relationship and can discourage collaboration.

6. Ask yourself a question: Do you want a collaborative, participatory relationship with your patient, or do you want to be authoritarian and paternalistic? The answer to that question should help you choose your preference in communication styles between the first and the alternate interaction.

SEE ONE, DO ONE, TEACH ONE

2

Before reading the interaction below, please consider the following topics:

Provider education
- Providers receive both academic and applied education
  - All interaction with or around students is an opportunity to illustrate effective health communication behaviors
- Humans cannot not communicate
  - All verbal and/or nonverbal behaviors communicate messages to receivers
  - Communication occurs whether intended by the sender or not

Building trust
- Providers need patients to trust them
  - To encourage information-sharing
  - To promote patient self-disclosure of personal information
  - To build interpersonal relationships
  - To attain goals

Communication is continuous
- Humans recall prior encounters in viewing current situation
  - You go to a restaurant and you expect to be greeted and seated
- Patients can be expected to remember how prior providers communicated with them
  - All providers will benefit from peers' use of effective interpersonal and health communication with patients

INITIAL INTERACTION

Role play and/or analyze the following communication exchange:

A student and healthcare provider stand next to a patient's bed in the Emergency Department. The patient, a 55-year-old man, is sitting up on the side of the bed, with a nasal canula providing oxygen. The student is holding a handful of blood-drawing supplies.

Provider:	"Okay, so we're going to draw some blood. Have you done this before?"
Student:	"No."
Provider:	"Great, I'll show you how, then you can do the next one, and then you'll be ready to teach your classmates how to do it."
Student:	"Sounds good."
Provider:	"The first thing you need to do is get all your equipment out where you can easily reach it, and then grab some gloves."
Mr. Johnson:	"What's going on?"
Provider:	"We're here to get some blood. It won't take very long and we'll be out of your way."
Mr. Johnson:	"Okay."
Provider:	"Now, the first thing you want to do is check the patient's bracelet, so you stick the right person. Then you need to put on a tourniquet above the elbow and get it tight enough to restrict blood flow from the veins, but you don't want to hurt him. I hate trying to feel for a vein with these gloves—it used to be so much easier before HIV—but sometimes you need to get the patient to open and close his fist and that will help make the vein pop-up better. Can you open and close your fist three or four times and then just keep a tight fist?"
Mr. Johnson:	"Okay."
Provider:	"Great, now feel this. Do you feel that lump there as you move your finger back and forth? Don't press hard; just very lightly run your finger back and forth."
Student:	"Is that it there?"
Provider:	"No, feel more over here."
Student:	"Oh, I feel that."
Provider:	"Okay, so next you want to be sure you wipe over the area with an alcohol pad, then get your needle and, with the bevel up, try to go in at about a 30-degree angle to the skin. Don't push in too far."

Mr. Johnson:	"Ow!"
Provider:	"Sorry, but don't move; we're almost done. Relax your hand and don't make a fist. When you think you're in the vein, try not to move the needle too much, but grab your first tube and push it onto the filler-needle firmly. You have to grip the plastic holder really tight, so you don't move the needle in the vein, or go through it, when you push the tube in. Let it fill up most of the tube, then pull it straight out, turn the tube up and down once or twice, then grab the next tube and fill it up. Got it?"
Student:	"Yeah, but how do you know when you're in the vein?"
Provider:	"You'll get used to the feel of it popping through the vein. Now, that's the last tube, so grab your 2x2 gauze pad, undo the tourniquet, and press down over where the needle goes into the skin, but not too hard—it will hurt. But as you pull the needle out, press down harder with the gauze pad. You can hold pressure for a few seconds and then ask the patient to hold it, or just put a piece of tape tightly across it, if the patient isn't on blood thinners, or is a bleeder. You ready to do the next one?"
Student:	"Sure."
Mr. Johnson:	"Not on me, okay?"

Discussion Questions

1. Besides the phlebotomy technique, what else did the student learn from this interaction? Why do you feel that way?

_____

_____

_____

_____

2. What verbal and nonverbal messages were communicated by the healthcare provider to Mr. Johnson?

_____

_____

_____

_____

3. How would you characterize the interaction that occurred in this scenario from the provider's, the patient's, and the student's perspectives? Be specific.

_____

_____

_____

_____

4. To enhance communication, how would you change the interaction?

_____

_____

_____

5. Discuss the nonverbal behaviors that you think communicated differently than intended?

_____

_____

_____

Interactive Activity

- Rewrite (individually or in a group) the interaction between the student, provider, and Mr. Johnson, and alter the verbal and nonverbal behaviors as needed to make the health communication exchange more effective for all participants.
- Compare your rewrite to the Alternate Interaction that follows.

Interaction Rewrite

_____

_____

_____

_____

_____

_____

_____

_____

_____

_____

_____

ALTERNATE INTERACTION

Insert your name and/or profession in the appropriate blanks below.

Provider: "Hi, Mr. Johnson. My name is _____, and I'm a _____."

Mr. Johnson: "Hi."

Provider: "This is _____, a _____ (profession) student. Is it all right with you if she/he observes while I get some blood?"

Mr. Johnson: "I don't care."

Provider: "I need to take some blood from your arm for some tests that are ordered. Would you like to lie down?"

Mr. Johnson: "Sure; I get a little light-headed around needles."

Provider: "No problem; we'll put the head of your bed up, so it will be almost like sitting up. Looks like you're having a bit of trouble breathing."

Mr. Johnson: "Yeah, I got this emphysema; too many cigarettes."

Provider: "Sorry, but I'm sure they'll get you feeling better. Now, is that more comfortable?"

Mr. Johnson: "It's okay—nothing's very comfortable when you can't breathe."

Provider: "Okay, so we're going to get started and I'll tell you everything I'm going to do before I do it."

Student: "How do you decide where to look for a vein?"

Provider: "The hand hurts more, so I try the elbow first. Make sure you lay out all the tubes, gauze pads, and alcohol wipes within easy reach. Then get gloved up. Mr. Johnson, I'm going to put a tourniquet on your arm; it may feel a bit tight, but I'll get it off as soon as I can. Would you mind opening and closing your fist a couple of times and then making a tight fist and holding it? Great, now I'm going to touch your arm and just feel for a vein."

Mr. Johnson: "No problem; I just don't want to watch."

Provider: "I don't blame you. Now I'm going to talk to _____ for a couple of minutes about what I'm doing here. So, I run my finger horizontally across the skin. I'm feeling for any bump or lump under the skin. There it is—can you feel that?"

Student: "I think so."

Provider: "Now we clean the area thoroughly with an alcohol wipe, and always let patients know before you stick them. Okay, Mr. Johnson, there's going to be a little stick. Try not to move your arm; I'll be as quick as I can."

Student: "You can use your other hand to squeeze my fingers if that will help."

Mr. Johnson:	"Thanks, I know I'm a 200-pound baby; I just always hate needles. Sorry if I'm squeezing too tightly."
Student:	"No problem."
Provider:	"Okay, Mr. Johnson, I'm getting the blood and it won't be much longer now. When you do the venipuncture, make sure the bevel is pointing up and at a 30–45-degree angle to the skin. Then just be sure you grip the plastic holder tightly, so it doesn't move the needle in the vein when you push the tube onto it. Let the tube fill up, then pull it out, turn it upside down a couple of times, and put it to the side, then get the next empty tube. Okay, Mr. Johnson, I'm all done and I'm going to release the tourniquet, then take the needle out and put a little pressure on it."
Mr. Johnson:	"Sounds good to me."
Student:	"Sounds good to me, too." (Mr. Johnson and the student laugh.)

Follow-up Discussion

1. How is this interaction different from the previous one? Is it more effective at communicating information?

   _____

   _____

   _____

2. Does the alternate scenario provide any communication that would enhance the patient's trust in the provider? If so, why? If not, why not?

   _____

   _____

   _____

3. How does the communication in this scenario differ from the initial example in terms of relationship-building? What specific behaviors support your response?

   _____

   _____

   _____

4. Does the student's offer to let the patient squeeze his/her fingers impact the interpersonal communication? If so, how? If not, why not?

_____

_____

_____

5. How might the alternate interaction impact the student's learning and his/her future health communication? Why do you feel that way?

_____

_____

_____

Key Points

1. Teaching students a clinical skill provides faculty an opportunity also to demonstrate or mentor effective communication skills.

2. Healthcare providers need to communicate with their patients. Interpersonal communication (between two people) requires trust and sharing of information. The more a provider can build a relationship with his/her patients, the easier it will be to gain their trust, gather information, educate, and empower them to make decisions about their health.

3. It takes little or no extra time to communicate effectively with a patient. However, the rewards for both the provider and patient, in terms of information-exchange, relationship-building, and decision-making, are critically important to successful outcomes.

4. Communication is continuous, so no matter what type of interaction healthcare providers have with patients, there is the potential to positively or negatively impact other current and future provider–patient interactions. Therefore, trying to enhance interpersonal communication behaviors and interpersonal relationships, even during a brief encounter like a blood draw, can have positive ramifications for future health communication.

THE BIOMEDICAL MODEL

3

Before reading the interaction below, please consider the following topics:

Biomedical model
- Approach to diagnosis and treatment that emphasizes a biological cause for illness
- Traditionally taught in medical and physician assistant programs
- Utilizes investigation to discover biological origin of patient's complaints

Nonverbal communication
- Relies on behaviors other than the spoken word
  - Complimenting
  - Contradicting
  - Accenting
  - Repeating

Relationship-building:
- Developed through interaction
- Requires work by both parties
- Based on relational prototypes
  - What is the provider's perception of an ideal patient?
  - What is the patient's perception of the ideal provider?

Developing trust
- Trust comes from
  - Effective interpersonal communication
  - Trustworthy behaviors of providers
  - Interpersonal relationship between provider and patient

INITIAL INTERACTION

Role play and/or analyze the following communication exchange:

Ms. Schwartz, a 33-year-old female, has been having stomach pains for the past week. She made an appointment with her provider and, after waiting for 20 minutes in the waiting room and for another 15 minutes in a thin gown and her underwear, the door opens suddenly. The provider, who Ms. Schwartz had seen only twice before, enters the room.

Provider:	"Hi. How are we doing today?"
Ms. Schwartz:	"I'm not feeling very well; it's cold in here, and you startled me."
Provider:	"Sorry, what's going on?"
Ms. Schwartz:	"About a week ago I started to notice a pain here in my stomach, just below my rib. I thought it would just go away, but—"
Provider:	"Did you have any nausea, vomiting, or diarrhea?"
Ms. Schwartz:	"No, not then, but later."
Provider:	"Did the pain go anywhere?"
	(The provider is now standing next to Ms. Schwartz and motions for her to lay back. Then the provider raises the gown, exposing her abdomen, panties, and legs. The provider begins palpating her abdomen.)
Ms. Schwartz:	"That hurts! But the pain doesn't go anywhere. I thought at first that it was just some indigestion, but when it kept coming back, a friend of mine thought it might be an ulcer."
Provider:	"Have you had an ulcer?"
Ms. Schwartz:	"No, but that's what Mary said it sounded like to her."
Provider:	"Well, I don't think it's an ulcer. I think you've got a little gastritis and you just need a couple of pills to help slow down your acid production, and you should be good as new in no time flat."
	(The provider moves toward the door and grabs the handle.)
Provider:	"Any questions? I'll leave a prescription with the receptionist. Go easy on the fried and greasy foods, stay away from aspirin or ibuprofen, and let us know if you have any more problems."
	(The provider turns the knob and rushes out the door.)

Discussion Questions

1. What is the biomedical model?

   _____

   _____

   _____

2. What communication behaviors in this interaction are typical of the biomedical model? Be specific.

   _____

   _____

   _____

3. How does the provider's reliance on the biomedical model impact the communication exchange and interpersonal relationship of these two individuals?

   _____

   _____

   _____

4. How would you describe Ms. Schwartz's description of her problem?

   _____

   _____

   _____

5. Describe how this exchange of information might have impacted the responses to the interaction for the provider, and for the patient.

   _____

   _____

   _____

6. What are some of the nonverbal behaviors and environmental factors that may be contributing to the patient's attitude, perceptions, and communication?

   _____

   _____

   _____

7. Identify four of the provider's communication behaviors that contributed negatively to the communication exchange.

   _____

   _____

   _____

Interactive Activity

- Rewrite (individually or in a group) the interaction between the provider and Ms. Schwartz, and alter the verbal and nonverbal behaviors as needed to make the health communication exchange more effective for both participants.
- Compare your rewrite to the Alternate Interaction that follows.
- What behaviors did you write that were similar to the example? Which were different?

Interaction Rewrite

ALTERNATE INTERACTION

A 33-year-old female is seated in a chair in an examination room; she is clothed and reading a magazine. There's a knock on the door and a provider in a white coat enters the room, goes over to the patient and shakes her hand. The provider then sits down on a rolling stool opposite the patient, at eye level, and makes eye contact as they speak.

Provider: "Hello, Ms. Schwartz. I'm sorry that you've been waiting; we had an emergency that delayed me a bit. I see from your chart that you told the nurse that your stomach has been bothering you. Can you tell me some more about that?"

Ms. Schwartz: "Well, about a week ago, I noticed a pain here in my stomach. It started around bedtime and I remember thinking that maybe it could have something to do with the sandwich I had for lunch that day—'cause it just didn't taste right. I got sick during the night and had diarrhea. It continued for several days. Now I don't have any more diarrhea, but I still have some pain here, but it's less than it was."

Provider: "It sounds like you've had a miserable week. What kind of a sandwich was it?"

Ms. Schwartz: "It's been an awful week. It was a chicken salad sandwich. Do you think that could've caused it?"

Provider: "Well, I can't be sure, but it sounds like things are getting better. But I'd like to examine your abdomen, check your stool for blood, and get a sample to do some laboratory tests for *Salmonella*, or other bacteria that can get into your system and cause pain and diarrhea. I'm going to have Sarah come in and help you get into a gown, then I'll come right back and we'll do the examination and the tests, and then we'll get you out of here. Do you have any questions before we proceed?"

Ms. Schwartz: "Do you think I need antibiotics? Am I contagious?"

Provider: "Those are both very good questions and, from your description, it sounds like things are improving, so I doubt you'll need antibiotics right now; but we'll know more after the examination and the tests come back. But I can tell you for sure that you're not contagious."

Ms. Schwartz: "I'm so glad. I've been afraid to even kiss my fiancée because I didn't want him to catch this."

Follow-up Discussion

1. Identify four nonverbal behaviors that you think are keys to enhancing the effectiveness of the interaction.

    _____

    _____

    _____

    _____

2. What is the benefit of the patient's narrative in the alternate example?

    _____

    _____

    _____

    _____

3. How does the communication in this scenario differ from the initial example in terms of relationship-building and trust? What specific behaviors support your response?

    _____

    _____

    _____

    _____

▐Key Points

1. Nonverbal behaviors communicate as much, or more than verbal messages:
   a. knocking on a door;
   b. unclothed versus clothed;
   c. eye contact;
   d. both patient and provider seated at eye level;
   e. provider not interrupting the patient;
   f. patient being allowed to tell her/his story (narrative);
   g. providing feedback to assure understanding.

2. Providers often state that they don't have time to listen to a patient's story, instead, they ask questions. This example demonstrates that more information can be gathered in a short amount of time by letting the patient tell her/his story. In addition, using questions to supply missing information requires less grilling and serves as feedback rather than quizzing behavior.

3. Relationship-building and -maintaining do not require lengthy discussions. However, they do require communication behaviors, verbal and nonverbal, that foster trust and encourage information-exchange and collaboration.

4. The biomedical model is designed to assure data gathering related to the signs and symptoms of disease. However, this specificity requires an emphasis on getting answers to certain key questions, and risks missing important information that could have been obtained by listening for more than just the biomedical information. Specifically, listening for psychological and/or sociological issues that might be affecting the patient's condition can provide added information that may be very important to the diagnosis.

THE BIOPSYCHOSOCIAL MODEL

4

Before reading the interaction below, please consider the following topics:

Biopsychosocial model
- Approach to diagnosis and treatment that explores problems as they relate to a variety of etiologies
  - Biological
  - Psychological
  - Sociological
- Typically taught in nursing and nurse practitioner programs

Hostile communication
- Can be marked by
  - Insults
  - Sarcasm
  - Contempt for other communicator
- Includes
  - Lack of eye contact
  - Minimal or no listening
  - Defensive response to questions or comments

Listening
- Hearing requires competent anatomy and physiology
- Listening is critical for effective communication
  - Requires conscious focus, assimilation, and assessment
  - Related to past experiences
  - Influenced by nonverbal cues

INITIAL INTERACTION

Role play and/or analyze the following example:

The patient is a 43-year-old male complaining of having a rash on his abdomen for a week. He presents to an outpatient clinic at a hospital with normal vital signs. After nearly 15 minutes, the provider enters the room.

Provider:	"Mr. Olecky? Hi, did I pronounce that right?"
Mr. Olecky:	"Yes, that's it; but I thought you'd forgotten about me. I've been waiting for a long time."
Provider:	"I'm sorry, but there are a lot of people to see. But now it's your turn. So tell me about your rash."
Mr. Olecky:	"Well, I got this rash on my stomach that's been there for about three days and I don't know why it's there." He pulls up his gown.
Provider:	"Hmm. Does it itch?"
Mr. Olecky:	"No, its just there and I don't know why."
Provider:	"Okay, can you tell me a bit more about what's going on in your life the last few days, what you've eaten, if you've got any new clothes, or changed soaps?"
Mr. Olecky:	"None of that."
Provider:	"Okay, do you have a rash anywhere else?"
Mr. Olecky:	"No. How many questions are you going to ask?"
Provider:	"It sounds to me like you are very annoyed. Is that all because of the wait?"
Mr. Olecky:	"Of course I'm annoyed. I've got this damn rash."
Provider:	"All right, so I'll get you a prescription for your rash."

Discussion Questions

1. What is the patient communicating to the provider?

_____

_____

_____

_____

2. How do you think the provider could have handled the situation differently?

_____

_____

_____

_____

3. How did the provider try to build a relationship with this patient?

_____

_____

_____

_____

4. In what ways did this provider use the biomedical model during the interaction?

_____

_____

_____

_____

5. What information do you think is missing from the evaluation of this patient?

_____

_____

_____

_____

6. How would you have handled this patient differently? Be specific.

_____

_____

_____

_____

Interactive Activity

- Rewrite (individually or in a group) the interaction between the provider and Mr. Olecky, and alter the provider's verbal and nonverbal behaviors as needed to make the health communication exchange more effective for both participants.
- How might you have dealt with the patient's hostility using a biopsychosocial approach?
- Compare your rewrite to the Alternate Interaction that follows.

Interaction Rewrite

ALTERNATE INTERACTION

Insert your name and/or profession in the appropriate blanks below.

The provider knocks on the door, enters the exam room, and shakes hands with the patient. The provider then sits down in a chair across from the patient.

Provider: "Hi, Mr. Olecky. I'm really sorry you had to wait. My name is _____, and I'm a _____. We've had a really busy morning and I do apologize; but now that I'm here, you have my undivided attention. Tell me about your rash."

Mr. Olecky: "Well, I started getting this rash about three days ago. It's only on my stomach. I tried to think if there was anything I ate different than usual, or if I'd changed soaps, or detergent; but I can't think of anything. I just need you to get me something so it goes away."

Provider: "I understand. No unusual foods, no new soaps or detergents. Any new clothes?"

Mr. Olecky: "No."

Provider: "Does it itch?"

Mr. Olecky: "No, it's just a red rash and I want it gone."

Provider: "Mr. Olecky, I know rashes can be very troubling, but you seem awfully upset. I wonder if your frustration is all related to the rash and your wait here, or if there's something else bothering you?"

Mr. Olecky: "I hate rashes, I hate waiting, and I hate my job. Don't you think those are enough reasons to be upset?"

Provider: "I agree, those are more than enough reasons. And since we've talked about the wait here and your rash, maybe we could spend a few minutes talking about your job."

Mr. Olecky: "What are you, a shrink? I came here for this rash."

Provider: "I completely understand, Mr. Olecky, and I am not a psychiatrist, but it's important to try and understand the cause of your rash. Sometimes rashes are caused by emotional issues, like problems or stress at home or at work. You mentioned work—do you want to discuss a bit more about what's going on there?"

Mr. Olecky: "Not a lot to discuss; my boss is a jerk."

Provider: "I'm sorry to hear that. I know how tough it can be when you work for someone who isn't very easy to get along with."

Mr. Olecky: "No, that's not it; I get along with him just fine—it's just that he's not very loyal, so I'm not sure where I stand with him. I've been working there for eight years and I don't know if I'll have a job next week or not. He just got rid of 10 people last month and no one knows who will be next."

Provider:	"That's awful. I can imagine that's pretty stressful, not knowing who will be out of a job and when."
Mr. Olecky:	"Yeah, it is, and it usually happens at the end of the month, so next week may find me without a job."
Provider:	"So, is your wife worried too?"
Mr. Olecky:	"Are you kidding? I haven't told her. Why would I want her worried about it?"
Provider:	"I see, so your wife doesn't know, which means you must be a bit worried about how she's going to react if she finds out, yes?"
Mr. Olecky:	"She's not going to find out!"
Provider:	"I don't mean to irritate you, but if you get laid off, she'll find out and she'll have to deal with it. But wouldn't it be easier on both of you if you could talk about it in advance and be able to discuss your concerns as well as some possible plans?"
Mr. Olecky:	"I don't know. I just don't want her worrying. And shouldn't we be talking about my rash?"
Provider:	"Well, I think we've been talking about your rash. I think your rash is related to all the stress you're under, and I think if you could talk about this with someone, like your wife or a therapist, you could probably reduce your stress and your rash would go away."
Mr. Olecky:	"Really?"
Provider:	"I think so, but I will give you the name of a dermatologist and a psychologist who are on-call today. I'd recommend that you follow-up with the dermatologist if the rash isn't better in a couple of days, and that you consider going to the psychologist just to talk. In the meantime, I'd suggest you have a discussion with your wife about work and your concerns. Don't you think she has a right to know—about your job and your stress?"
Mr. Olecky:	"I guess, but I've never been to a psychologist before."
Provider:	"Well, I think you'd find it a great opportunity to discuss your stress and your concerns about talking about it with your wife. I also believe that being able to talk with someone about all this will help you and your rash."
Mr. Olecky:	"Well, I certainly never thought that work could cause my rash, but it does make sense."

Follow-up Discussion

1. What are the communication differences in the two scenarios?

   _____

   _____

   _____

   _____

2. Why did the alternate scenario obtain different information for the provider to analyze than the first scenario?

   _____

   _____

   _____

   _____

3. How did the provider successfully diffuse the patient's anger about his waiting time?

   _____

   _____

   _____

   _____

4. Based solely on this interaction, do you think the rash is a primary or secondary
   diagnosis? Why?

   _____

   _____

5. How does the relationship between the provider and the patient develop in the
   second interaction versus the first one?

   _____

   _____

   _____

   _____

6. Where in the communication between the provider and patient does the provider
   move beyond the biological model? Give specific words or phrases.

   _____

   _____

   _____

   _____

Key Points

1. All too often in today's healthcare, patients become frustrated or agitated by things that are out of the provider's control, like the number of patients to be seen and the number of providers available to see patients, etc. However, in order to have an effective interpersonal communication exchange, providers need to find verbal and nonverbal behaviors to build a relationship, which require empathy, active listening, and trust.

2. While the biomedical model focuses on the biological causes for patient's complaints or problems, the biopsychosocial model explores how psychological and sociological aspects of the patient's life may be contributing to the complaint or problem.

3. By focusing on the patient's biological, psychological, and social history, providers can improve their data gathering and enhance their diagnostic assessment capabilities and information-sharing with patients.

4. Effective communication depends on both parties in an interaction sending, listening, assimilating, and providing feedback.

5. Remember that angry, frustrated, and/or hostile patients make communicating effectively much more difficult and, therefore, make accurate assessment and diagnosis problematic. As a result, providers need to work on minimizing the anger and frustration, so effective communication can occur.

Autonomy Is a Myth

5

Before reading the interaction below, please consider the following topics:

Phone conversations
- Limited communication effectiveness versus face-to-face interactions
  - Lack many nonverbal cues used for feedback
  - Can include uncertainty about the identity of other communicator

Denotative meaning
- Public or dictionary meaning of a word or phrase
  - Immunization means to prevent disease
- Providers and patients with appropriate health literacy can generally agree on the denotative meaning of words or phrases

Connotative meaning
- Personal or emotional meaning of a word or phrase
  - To one person, immunization means to travel
  - To another person, immunization means pain
- Providers and patients may have very different interpretations of words and phrases and their connotative meanings and, thus, risk miscommunication

Power
- Power is very similar to influence
- There are several types of power
  - Reward power
    - Getting a raise at work
  - Coercive power
    - Use of fear
  - Expert power
    - Healthcare providers, engineers, etc.

- Referent power
  - Charismatic leaders
- Legitimate power
  - Police officer or judge

INITIAL INTERACTION

Role play and/or analyze the following example.
Insert your name and/or profession in the appropriate blanks below.

The patient is a 25-year-old male complaining of having a pain in his lower back for one day. After talking with the patient and examining him, the provider ordered physical therapy (PT) evaluation and treatment. However, prior to approving the PT, the patient's health insurance case manager has called the provider with questions.

Provider:	"Hi. This is _____, and I'm the _____ taking care of Mr. Swan. How can I help you?"
Case Manager:	"I'm calling because I see you've ordered PT for Mr. Swan, and I wanted to know why you didn't give Ibuprofen and muscle relaxants a try first?"
Provider:	"Well, I saw the patient, I examined him, and I felt it would be best for his injury if he had PT at this point. I've been doing this for a while, and I think I know which patients will benefit from conservative treatment and which ones need more aggressive therapy."
Case Manager:	"I appreciate your experience, but our policy is that unless there is a neurological deficit, paresthesias, or weakness, we prefer anti-inflammatories and muscle relaxants. I see from your progress note that Mr. Swan had normal reflexes, equal strength in his legs, no change in his gait, no paresthesias, and no numbness. So we will not be covering the PT at this time. If you want to re-evaluate him in a week or two and see how he's doing, then we can reassess at that time."
Provider:	"You know I'm the person taking care of Mr. Swan?"
Case Manager:	"I do, and I'm the person who is deciding what will get paid for by Mr. Swan's insurance; so unless Mr. Swan wants to pay for it himself, he's going to need to give conservative treatment a chance. As I said, we'll be happy to re-evaluate if he's not better in a week or two."
Provider:	"I'm sure somebody will be contacting you."

Discussion Questions

1. How would you describe the key issues in this interaction?

   _____

   _____

   _____

2. How would you characterize the provider's tone in the conversation?

   _____

   _____

   _____

3. What are the problems for the provider?

   _____

   _____

   _____

4. What are the problems for the case manager?

   _____

   _____

   _____

5. How did the provider try to control the interaction?

   _____

   _____

   _____

6. Can you describe how interpersonal communication is impacted in a phone versus face-to-face interaction?

   _____

   _____

   _____

7. How would you have handled this situation differently?

   _____

   _____

   _____

8. In what ways do providers' perceptions of managed care potentially impact:
   a. their interactions with case managers?
   b. their treatment decisions?
   c. their interactions with patients?

   _____

   _____

   _____

   _____

   _____

Interactive Activity

- Rewrite (individually or in a group) the interaction between the provider and the case manager.
- How might you have used interpersonal communication to try and build a relationship with the case manager?
- Compare your rewrite to the Alternate Interaction that follows.

Interaction Rewrite

_____

_____

_____

_____

_____

_____

_____

_____

_____

_____

_____

_____

_____

_____

_____

_____

_____
_____
_____
_____
_____
_____
_____
_____
_____
_____
_____
_____
_____
_____
_____
_____
_____
_____
_____
_____
_____
_____

ALTERNATE INTERACTION

Insert your name and/or profession in the appropriate blanks below.

The provider answers the phone.

Provider:	"Hi."
Receptionist:	"Hi. I've got Mr. Swan's case manager, Ms. Tooma, on the phone for you."
Provider:	"Okay, transfer her back."
Provider:	"Hello, Ms. Tooma, I'm _____."
Case Manager:	"Hi, I'm looking at your order for Mr. Swan and I'm trying to understand why you ordered PT so quickly."

Provider: "I expected your call. I know it's a bit unusual to start PT so soon after an injury, but Mr. Swan has some extenuating circumstances."

Case Manager: "I didn't see anything about that in your progress notes; in fact, it sounds like a pretty mild lumbar strain from your notes."

Provider: "I think it is, but Mr. Swan is applying to be a fire fighter and he's got a fitness-for-duty exam in a week, so I was hoping that two or three PT sessions, combined with the Ibuprofen and cyclobenzaprine hydrochloride, would get him ready for the fitness test."

Case Manager: "I see, but we generally don't make exceptions so people can apply for a job."

Provider: "I understand, but I think the fire department uses you all for its insurance, so it wouldn't be like you were getting someone better so they could move to another plan. I just thought the expense for two or three sessions would likely save you all money because it would decrease the need for follow-up visits with me, etc."

Case Manager: "Okay, I'll approve three visits to PT, but unless there are other factors, I won't be able to approve any more than that, and I cannot start doing this for other patients."

Provider: "I completely understand. Thanks for your help."

Follow-up Discussion

1. What changed the outcome of the two interactions? Why?

_____

_____

_____

_____

_____

2. How does the provider's interpersonal communication in the alternate scenario influence the case manager's decision?

_____

_____

_____

_____

3. What role does critical thinking play in the provider's assessment of the telephone situation?

_____

_____

_____

4. In spite of the limited role nonverbal communication plays in telephone conversations, how do the provider's nonverbal behaviors in the alternate example help change the outcome?

_____

_____

_____

5. How does the provider demonstrate, via his/her interaction with the case manager, the use of the biopsychosocial model in communicating with Mr. Swan?

_____

_____

_____

6. What was the case manager's denotative (dictionary definition) meaning in his/her message to the provider?

_____

_____

7. How did the connotative (personal/emotional) meaning of the case manager's message differ from the denotative meaning?

_____

_____

_____

Key Points

1. Provider autonomy has been altered by managed care. Providers can choose to interact with health insurance or managed care employees in a hostile or defensive way, or they can try to build a relationship and use effective interpersonal communication.
2. By assessing the information needs of the case manager, the provider was able to communicate to her the data needed to accomplish the provider's goals.
3. Active listening skills include close attention to what the sender of messages says and how she/he says it, including the sender's nonverbal communication, and both the denotative and connotative meaning of the message.

BAD NEWS

6

Before reading the interaction below, please consider the following topics:

Family communication
- Most patients communicate with their family members about their health and the provider's findings, recommendations, and decision-making
- Providers frequently need to include, with the patient's approval, family members in conversations about the patient's health and treatment decisions
- For pediatric, elderly, or incapacitated patients, family members are often the major decision-makers, and must be consulted by the provider in addition to, or in lieu of, the patient

Empathic listening
- Allowing patients to express their problems and concerns
- Offering encouragement without judging
- Resulting from providers communicating their caring to patients
- Succeeding when patients are better able to understand and/or cope with their problems

Health literacy
- Requires using language choices that are appropriate for the education and comprehension level of the patient and/or family
  - Providers need to avoid technical jargon
  - Providers need to quickly assess the patient's and/or family's language skills and adapt their communication appropriately

INITIAL INTERACTION
Role play and/or analyze the following example:

The patient is an 88-year-old female, who is in the hospital after collapsing at home. Her daughter is at the bedside. The patient has regained consciousness, but is not oriented to time, place, or person. The provider enters the patient's room, greets the daughter, and goes immediately to the bedside and begins examining the patient.

Provider: "Hello."

Ms. Gunther: "How's my mom?"

Provider: "She's about the same as yesterday."

Ms. Gunther: "What does that mean? Is she going to be herself?"

Provider: "Didn't Dr. Donahue, the neurologist, talk with you?"

Ms. Gunther: "He said she'd had a stroke, but not much more."

Provider: "Yes, she had a CVA, and it's in the part of the brain that causes cognitive problems. Sometimes these things get a little better over time, but I would recommend you start looking for a long-term care facility where she can live and get some rehabilitation."

Ms. Gunther: "A CVA? How did this happen?"

Provider: "It looks like your mom had high blood pressure. Did she take her medicine and watch her diet?"

Ms. Gunther: "I guess. I don't live with her. She had a lot of pills that she took."

Provider: "Well, this usually happens because people don't take their medicines and their blood pressure gets too high."

Ms. Gunther: "So this is her fault? Is that what you're saying?"

Provider: "Not exactly, but clearly blood pressure needs to be kept under control in order to prevent a CVA."

Ms. Gunther: "Shouldn't her doctor have expected something like this?"

Provider: "Well, I don't think we can blame her doctor. But now she needs to be in a long-term care facility."

Ms. Gunther: "I don't understand—what's a long-term care facility?"

Provider: "It's like a nursing home. They have specialized equipment and staff to help her get better."

Ms. Gunther: "Okay, do I have some time to do all this?"

Provider: "Well, we can probably wait till Friday to discharge her."

Ms. Gunther:	"But that's only two days. I don't know if I can find a place by then; can't you keep her longer?"
Provider:	"No, I'm afraid it's not easy to keep people in the hospital these days, once they've reached the maximum care we can provide."
Ms. Gunther:	"This is terrible! You're throwing us out, and she's had a stroke?"
Provider:	"We're not throwing you out. But we do need for you to find her a bed in a long-term care facility ASAP, because Medicare isn't going to pay for her to be in a hospital after Friday. And I'm sure you don't want to have to pay for her to be here, if they will pay for her to be in a rehabilitation center."
Ms. Gunther:	"So, this is about money?"
Provider:	"Not exactly; but your mother's insurance, Medicare, only covers her for a certain length of stay in the hospital, then they expect her to go to a long-term facility for her care. I'm sorry, but I have to go see other patients. If you can start making arrangements, this will all work out."

Discussion Questions

1. How did the patient's diagnosis impact the interaction?

   _____

   _____

   _____

   _____

2. How would you characterize the provider's education of the family member about her mother's illness?

   _____

   _____

   _____

   _____

3. What are the health communication problems for the provider in this scenario?

   _____

   _____

   _____

   _____

4. How would you evaluate the effectiveness of this interaction from a provider's perspective?

_____

_____

_____

5. How would you evaluate the effectiveness of this interaction from the family member's perspective?

_____

_____

_____

6. In what way do the different perspectives impact the information-exchange between the two interactants?

_____

_____

_____

7. What do you think is the family member's perception of the provider and of the hospital?

_____

_____

_____

_____

8. How is the communication between the provider and family member likely to affect the family member's views of the patient's care?

_____

_____

_____

9. How would you have handled this situation differently?

_____

_____

_____

Interactive Activity

- Rewrite (individually or in a group) the interaction between the provider and the family member.
- How might you have used interpersonal communication to try and build a relationship with the family member?
- Compare your rewrite to the Alternate Interaction that follows.

Interaction Rewrite

_____

_____

_____

_____

_____

_____

_____

_____

_____

_____

_____

_____

_____

_____

_____

_____

_____

_____

_____

_____

_____

_____

_____

_____

_____

_____

_____

_____

_____

_____

_____

_____

ALTERNATE INTERACTION

The provider enters the hospital room and goes immediately to Ms. Gunther, who is seated near her mom's bed. The provider shakes hands with Ms. Gunther, and then moves to the bedside.

Provider: "Hi. If you don't mind, let me say hello to your mom and examine her, and then we can talk."

Ms. Gunther: "Okay, but I don't think she'll say much."

(The provider examines the patient.)

Provider: "Thanks for your patience. We can go to an office nearby to talk, if you'd prefer?"

Ms. Gunther: "No, I'd like to stay here with Mom, if you don't mind?"

Provider: "Not at all. We'll be talking about her, so I think it's great. I'm sure you're exhausted—have you gotten any sleep?"

(The provider pulls up a chair close to Ms. Gunther, sits down, and makes eye contact with her.)

Ms. Gunther: "Not much. She was always so full of life; it's just weird to see her like this. But thanks for asking; most everyone who comes in here is just so focused and in a hurry, they hardly notice I'm here."

Provider: "I'm sorry; I know how tough it can be to try and care for a family member and still take care of yourself."

Ms. Gunther: "You're right—it's not something we are very well prepared for. Can you tell me how she's doing and what I should be expecting?"

Provider: "Of course. First, let's talk about where we are now. As I think you've already discussed with Dr. Donahue, your mom had a stoke and that means that, for some period of time, part of her brain did not get as much blood and oxygen as it needed. When that happens, the part of the brain that doesn't get oxygen becomes injured and can't do the work it normally does."

Ms. Gunther: "I'm sorry about the tears, but I just can't figure out how she changed so quickly. She was so full of life one minute and unable to talk the next."

(The provider takes a tissue from a box next to the bed and hands it to the daughter.)

Provider: "I understand how confusing it can be. But there are two types of strokes: one occurs when the blood vessel in the brain gets blocked by a blood clot and oxygen can't get through to that part of the brain. The other type of stroke occurs when a blood vessel breaks in the brain, because of too much pressure, and blood leaks inside the skull; so there's both less oxygen going to one part of the brain, and leaked blood that's increasing pressure on the brain because it's in a closed space inside the skull."

Ms. Gunther: "That sounds awful. Which one did she have?"

Provider: "You may remember that we did an MRI when she came into the Emergency Department, and that showed that she had a blood vessel burst. But the next day an MRI showed that there wasn't any more blood inside the skull, so she didn't need surgery."

Ms. Gunther: "But what caused it to burst? She didn't fall or hit her head or anything."

Provider: "I know, but pressure builds up in our blood vessels, usually because of high cholesterol, or some other problem, and sometimes the veins or arteries just can't take the pressure any more and they burst. And when they do, it's like when you hit your arm and you don't cut your skin, but you get a bruise. The bruise is a collection of blood from a small blood vessel breaking under the skin when you hit your arm. The difference is: inside your skull, when a small blood vessel breaks, there's no place for the blood to go, so it presses on the brain."

Ms. Gunther: "But she didn't hit her head."

Provider: "I know. I was just trying to use that as an example in people with high blood pressure—did she have a history of high blood pressure?"

Ms. Gunther: "I think she did, and high cholesterol; but she was taking medicines."

Provider: "I know, but often the damage to the blood vessels has been done over time and, suddenly, one of them just gives out and bursts."

Ms. Gunther: "Wow, I thought if you were on medicine you were safe."

Provider: "Well, you're right. It does help to be on medicine, and it probably gave her a lot more quality time being on the medicine, but unfortunately, our bodies just can't last forever."

Ms. Gunther: "I know, and we've been really lucky to have Mom be so healthy for so long; but I'm not ready to lose her yet."

(The provider reaches over and touches Ms. Gunther on the arm.)

Provider: "I'm sorry, I know this is difficult. But this is very early in your mom's recovery, so we don't know how much of her old self she'll get back. But that's what we need to discuss next."

Ms. Gunther: "Thanks for talking to me. I'm just glad she's here."

Provider: "You're welcome, and being here is what we need to talk about now. Your mom is going to need rehabilitative care where the therapists can help get back some of her thinking and speaking skills. She'll also need some physical therapy to make sure her muscles stay toned up while she's recovering."

Ms. Gunther:	"Does Medicare pay for that?"
Provider:	"Yes, I'm pretty sure they do, but not in the hospital. The next step is for you to meet with our social worker, and she'll have lots more information about potential facilities and Medicare coverage. We need to find a place that works for you and that offers the kind of rehabilitative therapy your mom needs."
Ms. Gunther:	"You mean she has to leave here?"
Provider:	"Yes, I'm afraid that once we get patients stabilized, they have to go to a facility that is intended to take care of them long-term. That's not what we do here. We take care of patients' urgent health problems, but for more chronic or prolonged care, there are better places than a hospital."
Ms. Gunther:	"Well, it seems really fast to get her out of here; but I've heard that women are sent home a lot quicker after having a baby than they used to be."
Provider:	"That's true, and you've probably heard in the news lately about the increased risk of infection the longer patients are in the hospital, so our goal is to treat people and get them to the next appropriate place for care as soon as possible."
Ms. Gunther:	"So what do I have to do and by when?"
Provider:	"You don't have to do anything. I'll write an order and the social worker will come see you and bring you information on the long-term care facilities near your home. Then you can contact the one that you prefer and see if they have a bed available for your mom. When you find one that does, the social worker will try to schedule a transfer on Friday, and I'll be around later to discuss how that happens and to answer any questions."
Ms. Gunther:	"Thanks so much. I'm nervous about all this, but it sounds like you know what you're doing and you've done this before, so that makes me feel a bit better."
Provider:	"I'm glad we got to visit and you're right, we do this all the time and it works really well for patients and their families. But I'll stop by later and see how you're doing and if you have any more questions."

Follow-up Discussion

1. How would you compare this interaction with the previous one?

_____

_____

_____

_____

2. How does the provider's interpersonal communication in the alternate scenario influence the family member's communication?

_____

_____

_____

_____

3. What role does listening play in the outcome of this conversation?

_____

_____

_____

_____

4. How did nonverbal communication impact the alternate discussion from the family member's perspective?

_____

_____

_____

_____

5. How does the provider use his/her understanding of the sociological aspects of healthcare to help communicate the patient's situation and future needs or status?

_____

_____

_____

6. How does the provider demonstrate her/his assessment of the family member's health literacy in the language choices made in the alternate scenario versus the initial one?

_____

_____

_____

7. Where in the alternate scenario do you see the provider using interpersonal communication to build a relationship with Ms. Gunther?

_____

_____

_____

Key Points

1. Patients and/or family members often do not understand why patients are discharged from the hospital more quickly than they expect.
2. By understanding patients' and family members' concerns about discharges, providers can assess, in advance, the content and interpersonal communication that will be needed to effectively share information and enhance decision-making.
3. Empathic listening requires individuals in an interpersonal relationship or interaction to try and understand the patient's or family member's situation and concerns, and empathize with them. By doing so, the provider can communicate her/his understanding and provide feedback that will help build trust and enhance their relationship.
4. By taking time and listening, as well as speaking, potentially bad news can be communicated in a way that encourages discussion and information-sharing, rather than frustration and verbal aggression.
5. Health literacy is an important component of effective health communication. Providers must recognize the education level of the patient and/or family member, and use language choices that are appropriate for the other communicator's understanding. In particular, providers should avoid technical jargon, like medical vocabulary or terminology, in communication with patients and family members.

CLOSINGS

7

Before reading the interaction below, please consider the following topics:

Closing conversations
- How providers close an interaction with a patient has a major impact on the patient's perception of the provider
  - Providers can choose to close a conversation by controlling the situation and shutting off any further communication
  - Provider and patient can mutually agree that all information has been exchanged and understood, and no questions remain

Nonverbal behaviors
- Frequently are more trusted by receivers than verbal messages
- Providers need to analyze their nonverbal behaviors to assure they are not contradicting their verbal messages with their nonverbal cues

Power sharing
- Providers choose how to use their power
  - Expert power is derived from the providers' professional roles and education
    - Expert power can be used to inform and empower patients
    - Expert power can be used to control information-sharing
    - Expert power can be used in an authoritarian or paternalistic manner

INITIAL INTERACTION

Role play and/or analyze the following example.
Insert your name and/or profession in the appropriate blanks below.

John Loomis is a 28-year-old CEO of an internet company. He's come to a provider's office complaining of a two-week history of fever, malaise, and fatigue. The patient is seated on the examination table in his underwear and a patient gown. The provider enters the room, moves to the countertop and places the chart down on it, then starts looking through it.

Provider:	"Hi. I'm _____, a _____. What brings you here today?"
Mr. Loomis:	"I came in my Lexus."
Provider:	"That's funny. I meant, what problem are you here for?"
Mr. Loomis:	"I wasn't trying to be funny. I've been having a fever for a couple of weeks. I get tired a lot and I need to be done with this."
Provider:	"How high is your fever?"
Mr. Loomis:	"I don't know—I don't take it. I feel hot and I get all sweaty. But mostly, I'm tired a lot and that's not me."
Provider:	"Have you had a sore throat or a cough?"
Mr. Loomis:	"No, nothing except the fever and being tired."
Provider:	"How about a rash?"
Mr. Loomis:	"Nope."
Provider:	"Any pains in your abdomen, change in your bowel habits, or burning when you urinate?"
Mr. Loomis:	"No, no, no."
Provider:	"Any discharge from your penis?"
Mr. Loomis:	"God no!"
Provider:	"Any drug use?"
Mr. Loomis:	"You mean besides Ibuprofen? No."
Provider:	"Any tick bites?"
Mr. Loomis:	"No. Wouldn't it be easier for me to just fill out a checklist?"
Provider:	"Sorry, but the list would be different for everyone, depending on their problems and symptoms. We're just about done with the questions. Have you traveled abroad recently?"
Mr. Loomis:	"I work on the internet; I don't travel out of my office if I can help it."
Provider:	"Okay, I'm going to examine you, and then we'll get some tests."
	(The provider does a physical examination, picks up the chart, and grabs the door knob.)

> **Provider:** "I've got the information I need. We'll get some blood tests, a chest X-ray, and a few other tests. They'll give you an appointment for Friday, and we can talk about the results then. Any questions?"
>
> **Mr. Loomis:** "Now you're kidding, right?"

Discussion Questions

1. How did the provider signal she/he was ready to close the conversation (verbally and nonverbally)?

   _____

   _____

   _____

2. How would you describe the interaction from the patient's and the provider's perspectives?

   _____

   _____

   _____

   _____

3. How did the provider use interpersonal communication to build trust and credibility with the patient?

   _____

   _____

   _____

4. What do you think was Mr. Loomis's perception of the provider?

   _____

   _____

   _____

   _____

5. How do you close conversations, especially with patients or their family members?

   _____

   _____

   _____

6. Which do you think—nonverbal or verbal behaviors—communicate more effectively your intention to close a conversation?

_____

_____

_____

7. Discuss, for each of these behaviors, how they illustrate and/or demonstrate the power or powerless aspects of the provider or patient, and why:
   a. standing and talking to a seated patient;
   b. dressed provider and undressed patient;
   c. lack of details about the reasons for the tests;
   d. minimal opportunity for the patient to provide feedback;
   e. provider asking for questions with his/her hand on door knob;
   f. reading the chart while talking to the patient.

_____

_____

_____

_____

_____

Interactive Activity

- Rewrite (individually or in a group) the interaction between the provider and the family member.
- How might you have used nonverbal communication specifically in your interpersonal communication to try and build a relationship with Mr. Loomis?
- Compare your rewrite to the Alternate Interaction that follows.

Interaction Rewrite

_____

_____

_____

_____

_____

_____

_____

_____

_____

ALTERNATE INTERACTION

The provider knocks on the door, then enters the examination room; the patient is dressed in a gown and sitting on the examination table. The provider goes directly to a rolling chair near the table, sits down, and makes eye contact with the patient.

Provider: "Hello again. So we talked about your fever and your fatigue, your past medical history, your family medical history, and your work and social life. Now I need to examine you. But first, was there anything you thought of while you were changing that we didn't discuss and that you think we should?"

Mr. Loomis: "Well, I'm sure it's not important, but I did remember that about three weeks ago I went to a friend's house for dinner and they had a sick kid, but he was in bed and I wasn't around him. Plus I think it was a strep. throat or something."

Provider: "And your fever's started about a week after that?"

Mr. Loomis: "Yeah, but that's all I forgot to tell you . . . You don't think it means anything do you?"

Provider: "Well, I'm not sure, but the more information we have the better it is. I planned to test you for Epstein Barr Virus: it causes mononucleosis and it's possible you could have gotten it there, but it also could be lots of other things as well."

Ms. Loomis: "You mean a guy my age can get mono.? I thought that was just in teenagers."

Provider: "More common in teens, but also happens to folks your age. So, I'm going to do your examination, then we'll get your tests done, and we'll sit down and talk for a bit."

Ms. Loomis: "Sounds like a plan."

(The provider finished the examination; the patient had blood tests, a purified protein derivative or TB test placed, and a chest X-ray. After dressing, the patient went to the provider's office and sat in a chair next to the desk.)

Mr. Loomis: "I thought you'd have a bigger office." (They both laugh.)

Provider: "Yeah, I thought it would be bigger too. Now, I want to discuss what we know and what we want to find out. Do you have a couple more minutes?"

Mr. Loomis: "Yeah, that's what I came here for."

Provider: "Great! Your symptoms: intermittent fever and fatigue over a prolonged period can be caused by a number of viruses or other conditions. With your history and symptoms, it seems very likely that this will have a viral origin, like mononucleosis, or cytomegalovirus (CMV). CMV is caused by a type of herpes virus, like the one that causes cold sores."

Mr. Loomis: "Wow, that's funny you mention that because my girlfriend had a cold sore a couple of weeks ago."

Provider:	"So, we're testing your blood for all those things, plus some other diseases that I don't think you have, like leukemia and HIV. As I said, you don't have any symptoms or signs from my physical examination of those, but just to be thorough, we want to check for them. Also the test on your arm is to rule out TB (tuberculosis). Again, your only real symptom for TB is your fever; you said you don't have night sweats, daily coughing, a history of recent travel to, or work in, a high-risk TB area. And the chest X-ray is just to rule out any surprises, and I looked at it already and it looks normal. Plus the radiologist will also look at it, and if there's anything different in the interpretation I'll contact you, but I really don't expect that to happen."
Mr. Loomis:	"WOW! So let me ask: you think I should be worried about having cancer or HIV? Should I tell my girlfriend to get checked?"
Provider:	"No, I certainly don't think you have cancer or HIV. And we'll have the results back in two days, so I wouldn't recommend that your girlfriend be tested. But I do want you to know what I'm ruling out with my interview, examination, and tests. In my opinion, you most likely have a viral infection, but because you've had these symptoms for a while, we need to make sure it's not something else. But I don't think its cancer or anything else except a virus, like mono."
Mr. Loomis:	"Okay, that sounds good. I've got to tell you, it's going to be a long couple of days."
Provider:	"I understand and I wish I could completely allay your concerns, but I've told you what I think and why, and I'll be happy to talk with you if you have more questions when you get home. But you can expect a call from me as soon as we have the results back."
Mr. Loomis:	"That's great, and I want to thank you for explaining this to me."
Provider:	"I'm glad we could talk, but I want to see if you have any more questions, or if there's anything else you want to discuss?"
Mr. Loomis:	"Nope, I think you've done it; but I'll be happy when I get your call and we have a definite answer for this."
Provider:	"Me too, and it would be a good idea for you to actually take your temperature every time you feel hot, and keep a little diary with the day and time and temperature, so you can tell me about it when we talk on the phone. Also, you should take some Ibuprofen, with food, for any temperatures above 100 degrees."
Mr. Loomis:	"Okay. I've never kept a diary before, so that'll be new." (They both laugh.)
Provider:	"Just jot down the date and time for any temperatures above 100, so it won't be a lot of work. Any other questions I can answer?"
Mr. Loomis:	"Nope. I'll talk to you soon."
	(The provider stands up and extends a hand to the patient.)
Provider:	"I'll be in touch as soon as I hear anything. Try not to worry; it will only increase your fatigue."
Mr. Loomis:	"Got it! Thanks again."

Follow-up Discussion

1. How would you compare this interaction with the previous one?

   _____

   _____

   _____

2. How does the provider's interpersonal communication in the alternate scenario impact the information gathering and the patient's responses?

   _____

   _____

   _____

3. How does the closing in this conversation potentially affect the patient's attitude toward the provider?

   _____

   _____

   _____

4. How did the nonverbal communication surrounding the closing of the alternate conversation change your perception of the provider?

   _____

   _____

   _____

5. How do you close conversations with patients?

   _____

   _____

   _____

6. How does the closing in the alternate scenario illustrate a power sharing between the interactants?

   _____

   _____

   _____

7. How did the discussion in the provider's office change the closing?

   _____

   _____

   _____

8. If you were the patient, which of the two scenarios would you prefer for a closing and why?

_____

_____

_____

Key Points

1. Closings of interactions require effective nonverbal behaviors as well as verbal communication.
2. Power can be communicated nonverbally as well as verbally.
3. Providers need to know how they close conversations with patients, family members, and peers.
4. Feedback, seeking questions from receivers, or asking them to restate what they heard you say, is an important way for providers to assess receivers' understanding in conversations. However, feedback does much more. Feedback lets the receiver know that you are interested in having them ask questions, and that you want to do all you can to minimize confusion or miscommunication.
5. Nonverbal behaviors can be used to communicate to patients that a provider wants to have a collaborative relationship and not an authoritarian, paternalistic relationship. For example, some nonverbal behaviors that communicate equality between interactants include:
   a. providers sitting when talking with a seated patient or family member;
   b. patients being dressed except during the actual examination;
   c. providers not asking questions while their behaviors indicate they are ready to depart the room;
   d. providers' offices arranged so there are no obstacles between provider and patient while talking;
   e. providers using feedback to clarify what patients or family members communicate, and to demonstrate that they are listening and assimilating the information they are being given.

FOLLOW-UP

8

Before reading the interaction below, please consider the following topics:

Interpersonal relationships
- Rely on effective interpersonal communication
- Work best when provider and patient share common goals
- Increase trust and information-sharing among communicators

Communication context
- The settings where communication occurs
- Impact interactions and interpersonal communication
  - Communication in the Emergency Department is generally different from conversations in a provider's office
  - Health communication via the phone or e-mail are different from face-to-face interactions

INITIAL INTERACTION

Role play and/or analyze the following example:

Clara Jennings is a 42-year-old woman, who works in a bakery. She hurt her back lifting racks of bread, and has been seen at the Occupational Health clinic for the past two weeks. She comes in today with continued pain in her lumbar area and paresthesias in her right leg and foot. The provider opens the door, enters the room, and rests the patient's chart on the countertop across the room from the chair where the patient is seated.

Provider:	"Hi, Clara. What seems to be the problem today?"
Ms. Jennings:	"It's the same problem that I've been seeing you for, for the last few weeks: my back—remember?"
Provider:	"Oh, yes, I meant, how is your back?"
Ms. Jennings:	"It's not very good. It hurts in the daytime and it hurts at night, and now the pain is going down into my leg."
Provider:	"How's PT?"
Ms. Jennings:	"What's that?"
Provider:	"You know, physical therapy."
Ms. Jennings:	"I haven't had any of that. Your secretary said they'd call, but so far—no call."
Provider:	"Well that's not good; I would have hoped you would have been to a couple of treatments by now. Stand up and show me how far you can bend over."
	(The patient stands, bends at the hips to about 45 degrees and stops.)
Ms. Jennings:	"It hurts about there."
Provider:	"Does the pain go anywhere?"
Ms. Jennings:	"Yeah, it goes down my butt cheek into my leg and makes my foot tingle."
Provider:	"Okay, stand up straight, don't move your feet, and turn one way as far as you can."
Ms. Jennings:	"That's it."
Provider:	"Does that make it hurt in your leg?"
Ms. Jennings:	"No."
Provider:	"Good, now turn the other way as far as you can; does that hurt or go anywhere?"
Ms. Jennings:	"No."
Provider:	"Okay, good. Now walk toward me on your heels. Any pain?"
Ms. Jennings:	"No."

Provider:	"Can you lie down on the table? Now I'm going to raise your legs and tell me if it hurts at all."
Ms. Jennings:	"That hurts in my back."
Provider:	"Okay, but only the right leg makes it hurt?"
Ms. Jennings:	"Yes."
Provider:	"Okay, so sit up and let your legs hang down, and I'll check your reflexes."
Ms. Jennings:	"So when am I going to start feeling better?"
Provider:	"Once we can get you some PT, you'll start feeling better. So, how's work going?"
Ms. Jennings:	"I can't do my job, because I can't bend, so they sent me home."
Provider:	"So, you're not working?"
Ms. Jennings:	"They said they don't have any light duty. So, I need to get better, 'cause I need to go back to work."
Provider:	"All right, I'll have the receptionist check on the PT, and we'll see you back next week."

Discussion Questions

1. What is your impression of the patient's reaction to the provider not remembering her back problem?

   _____

   _____

2. How did the context of the interaction, a worker's compensation injury, impact the conversation?

   _____

   _____

3. How would you have handled the patient's delayed physical therapy evaluation and treatment?

   _____

   _____

4. What do you think was Ms. Jennings' perception of the provider, and why?

   _____

   _____

   _____

5. In what way did the fact that this was a follow-up visit alter the exchange of information between the provider and patient?

_____

_____

_____

6. Because this was a follow-up for a specific worker's compensation injury, how do you think that affects the interpersonal relationship between the provider and the patient?

_____

_____

_____

7. What impact do you think the provider's responsibility to both employee and employer has on the provider's interaction with the patient?

_____

_____

_____

Interactive Activity

- Rewrite (individually or in a group) the interaction between the provider and the patient.
- How would you alter the outcome of this scenario in terms of getting her a physical therapy appointment?
- Compare your rewrite to the Alternate Interaction that follows.

Interaction Rewrite

_____

_____

_____

_____

_____

_____

_____

_____

_____

_____

ALTERNATE INTERACTION

Insert your name and/or profession in the appropriate blanks below.

The provider enters the room and goes over and shakes the woman's hand. The provider pulls a rolling chair over and sits next to the woman, who is clothed and seated in a chair.

Provider: "Hello, Ms. Jennings. How is your back today?"

Ms. Jennings: "It's not so good."

Provider: "I'm sorry; I thought with the physical therapy and restricted work, it would be better. Tell me about your week."

Ms. Jennings: "Well, first, I never got the physical therapy. I called and they said they'd call back, but they never did. And now, it's not just my back hurting, the pain goes down the back of my leg into my foot. It feels like my foot's asleep. And work's not helping; they don't have me lifting, but I have to count loaves on racks, so there's a lot of up and down and twisting and turning. I go home and I'm in pain, and they don't care."

Provider: "I'm very sorry about the confusion with physical therapy, and I'm really sorry to hear about your back feeling worse. So when you bend over, is that when you feel the pain in your leg and foot?"

Ms. Jennings: "Yes, but not every time."

Provider: "Got it. Now when you say pain—I want to make sure I understand exactly what you mean—is this a sharp pain, or is it more like a needles-and-pins feeling?"

Ms. Jennings: "It's needles-and-pins; the sharp pain is in my back, more on the right side here and then down into my right leg."

(The provider palpates the patient's lumbar area.)

Provider: "Okay, so you may remember that we talked before about how muscles can spasm, trap a nerve, and cause your pain in the back?"

Ms. Jennings: "Yeah."

Provider: "Well, if it traps the sciatic nerve—that's the nerve that goes down through your butt and triggers the nerves in your leg and foot—the nerve gets pinched by the muscle, and then you get the needles-and-pins feeling in your leg and foot. But the other thing that can cause that feeling is if the nerve is getting caught by a disc in your spine that's out of place. So what we have to do is find out if your discs in your lower back, that control the nerves to your legs and feet, are in alignment or not. So to do that we need to get an MRI. Does that make sense?"

Ms. Jennings: "I'm not sure."

Provider: "I understand; it's a lot of information. Can you tell me what you heard me say?"

Ms. Jennings: "Well, you said that a nerve in my back, sci-something, is the reason why I have the pain in my leg and foot. But you said that it could be caused by a muscle pinching it, or it could be caused by a messed up disc in my back. I'm not sure what else you said."

Provider: "You did really good. The last thing I mentioned was that we need to do an MRI—it's a very special X-ray that looks at the discs in your back and can tell us if they are out of alignment; and if they are, they are likely pushing on a nerve. Does that make more sense?"

Ms. Jennings: "Yes. I've heard of MRIs, but I've never had one."

Provider: "Well, the good news is that they don't hurt; you just have to lie still for a few minutes and that's all there is to it. But if the MRI shows a problem with one of your discs, we'll have you see a neurosurgeon."

Ms. Jennings: "I'll need surgery?"

Provider: "Probably not; even if you have a disc that is causing your problem, it can often be relieved by physical therapy, rest, and Ibuprofen. But we like to have a neurosurgeon evaluate you, just to see if there are any other treatment plans that they want us to try. But, let's not get ahead of ourselves; for now, it still sounds like its muscular and we're going to proceed with the physical therapy, because you'd need that regardless of whether it's a muscle or disc that's pushing on your nerve."

Ms. Jennings: "But I can't get physical therapy."

Provider: "Well, let's see if I can help."

(The provider goes to the phone on the wall and dials.)

Provider: "Hi. This is _____, a _____ at Occupational Health, and I'm calling about Clara Jennings, a patient I ordered a PT evaluation and treatment for, about a week and a half ago. She's been unable to get an appointment, so I was hoping that I could get one scheduled now, since she's in for an examination today and really needs to get some PT started."

(The provider turns to Ms. Jennings.)

Provider: "Do you want to come talk to them; they can schedule an appointment while we're on the phone, so why don't you see what day and time works best for you."

Ms. Jennings: "Sounds good to me."

Follow-up Discussion

1. How would you compare this interaction with the previous one?

_____

_____

_____

2. How does the provider's interpersonal communication in the alternate scenario impact the information exchange?

    _____

    _____

    _____

3. How does the provider's request for a narrative: "tell me about your week?" contribute to, or detract from, the provider's information-gathering as compared to the first example?

    _____

    _____

    _____

4. What nonverbal communication behaviors do you think impacted the patient's perception of the provider?

    _____

    _____

    _____

    _____

5. What do you think the provider's action of calling the PT Department in the patient's presence communicated about the provider?

    _____

    _____

    _____

6. How is power illustrated differently in the two scenarios?

    _____

    _____

    _____

7. Why do you think the provider in scenario number two discussed the diagnostic tests, possible results, and various treatment plans with the patient before she/he examined the patient?

    _____

    _____

8. How does the context (follow-up worker's compensation injury) of this communication potentially impact the style and content of the provider–patient interaction?

    _____

    _____

    _____

Key Points

1. Follow-up visits, by their very nature, are different from a communication perspective because they are even more a continuous relationship than a once-a-year, or an acute visit. Patients are more likely to bring an expectation that the provider remembers, or at least has read about, the prior visit(s) before speaking with the patient.

2. Power can be communicated in a variety of ways, and power-sharing can be illustrated through actions such as taking responsibility for helping a patient instead of minimizing the problem or passing it off to someone else.

3. Allowing patients to "tell their stories" through a brief narrative accomplishes several important goals for both the patient and the provider:
   a. patient feels like she/he gets to communicate what she/he feels is important, in an open-ended manner;
   b. provider gets to hear more information than what is possible through closed-ended questions and answers;
   c. provider usually doesn't need to interrupt as much, so is less paternalistic or authoritarian;
   d. patient gets a chance to include pertinent psychological and sociological aspects of the situation, not just the biological issues;
   e. provider may learn something pertinent to the diagnosis.

4. Asking the patient to reiterate "what she/he heard" encourages the patient to provide feedback that the provider can use to assess understanding, assimilation, or miscommunication. However, it's important that the patient be asked what she/he heard and not "what I said," because the latter is more authoritarian and implies that the provider never misspeaks. "What you heard," on the other hand, implies that there may be some miscommunication, but does not imply anyone is at fault.

5. Explaining to patients what the plan is, and why, should not be seen as always a concluding or closing event. In some cases, especially in follow-up visits where the patient and provider have previously discussed various aspects of the patient's illness or injury, the important consideration is that the patient is well-informed and understands what the provider is thinking, and why, and the patient is then empowered to make decisions about his/her treatment. Because the discussion of next steps and the treatment plan have been done, traditionally, at the end of an interaction between a provider and patient, this should in no way limit the discussion at any appropriate point in the interaction. In many instances, making the patient wait until the end of the examination may create more tension and anxiety, which could have been minimized or alleviated by a discussion earlier in the interaction.

I'VE GOT THE LICENSE, SO WE'RE DOING IT MY WAY

9

Before reading the interaction below, please consider the following topics:

Leadership communication
- Needed to influence others
- Providers frequently are expected to take on leadership roles with peers and subordinates, and also with patients and family members
  - As department or team leaders
  - In crises
  - When difficult decisions need to be made
- Provider's personality can impact others' perceptions of him/her as a leader

Negotiation
- Providers need to understand the patients' and/or family members' goals and needs
- Requires a free flow of information between provider and patient/family member(s)
- Providers should strive to attain collaborative goals
  - All parties need to be well informed
  - Information-sharing is critical
- When collaboration is not possible, compromising strategy is needed
  - Provider and patient will need to modify priorities to reach a mutually desired outcome

INITIAL INTERACTION

Role play and/or analyze the following example:

Two healthcare providers from different professions are working on the same team, caring for a patient who is elderly, has pneumonia, and is having difficulty breathing. The senior ranking person wants to intubate the patient in her bed on the medical–surgical floor. The junior ranking provider disagrees with the plan, and the two of them are having a discussion at the patient's bedside.

Provider A: "Look, she just needs to be intubated, then we'll move her to the ICU."

Provider B: "She needs to be in the ICU, that's the policy."

Provider A: "We've got respiratory techs, a nurse, and me here—we don't need anything else, except the intubation supplies and the ambu bag."

Provider B: "I don't agree. They have better monitoring equipment and are set up to do this routinely—we're not. That way she can go right on the ventilator instead of us bagging her till we get there. She's breathing; her blood pressure and pulse are fine, and it's less than five minutes from here to the ICU. Let's just move her instead of wasting time discussing it."

Provider A: "This is not open for discussion. I've got the license, so we're doing it my way."

Provider B: "Well, you may have the license, but I am taking the patient." (Provider B unplugs the oxygen from the wall and connects it to a portable tank, then unplugs the bed and pushes it out the door and down the hall, with Provider A and the rest of the team following.)

Note: The patient was successfully intubated five minutes later in the ICU without sequelae. Provider B was fired for not following Provider A's order. Provider B sued the hospital for wrongful termination.

Discussion Questions

1. What are your thoughts on this interaction, and on the providers' behaviors?

_____

_____

_____

_____

2. How do you think leadership communication impacted the outcome in this scenario?

   _____

   _____

   _____

   _____

3. What do you think is the role power plays in the communication of each provider's position?

   _____

   _____

   _____

   _____

4. Do you think either provider was using interpersonal communication skills to try and build a relationship? If so, why? If not, why not?

   _____

   _____

   _____

   _____

   _____

5. How do you think the setting for this interaction (at the bedside) potentially impacts the decision-making and communication?

   _____

   _____

   _____

   _____

6. What nonverbal communication behaviors do you think are most effective and why?

   _____

   _____

   _____

   _____

7. How would you evaluate the negotiation in this scenario, based on the organization's policy versus Provider A's decision to intubate on the floor?

   _____

   _____

   _____

   _____

Interactive Activity

- Rewrite (individually or in a group) the interaction between the two providers.
- How would you alter this interaction to improve the communication effectiveness and relationship-building between the two providers?
- Compare your rewrite to the Alternate Interaction that follows.

Interaction Rewrite

_____

_____

_____

_____

_____

_____

_____

_____

_____

_____

_____

_____

_____

_____

_____

_____

_____

_____

_____

_____

_____

_____

_____

_____

_____

_____

_____

_____

_____

_____

_____

_____

_____

_____

ALTERNATE INTERACTION

Provider A (senior ranking provider) and Provider B (different profession and junior ranking to Provider A) are in the meeting room off the nurse's station on the medical–surgical floor.

Provider A: "I understand that the hospital's policy is not to intubate on the floor unless it's a cardiac or respiratory arrest, but I don't want to take the chance that she arrests along the way; then we've got a code in the elevator or in the hall."

Provider B: "I share your concern, but if she has a cardiac arrest during the tubing, we've got the same problem in her room."

Provider A: "She's not going to arrest during the tubing."

Provider B: "Let's do this: let's call the house supervisor and get a third opinion."

Provider A: "We could be done already. But I guess another few minutes hopefully won't matter."

Supervisor: "I think you both make some really good points and I can understand each of your positions. How about if we hold the elevator, and we all go together."

Provider A: "I know you want to follow policy, and I still think we could intubate her first, but let's move her and hope for the best. I just want to get her tubed and on a ventilator."

Provider B: "Sounds good to me."

Supervisor: "Thanks. I've got some help gathered up, and we'll do this right now and get her upstairs and tubed."

Follow-up Discussion

1. What are some of the key differences between the two scenarios?

_____

_____

_____

_____

2. How does leadership by each member of the interaction impact the final outcome?

_____

_____

_____

_____

3. In what way does power shift in the second scenario compare with the first?

_____

_____

_____

4. What nonverbal communication behaviors do you think impacted the outcome of this interaction?

_____

_____

_____

_____

5. How did the use of a third person for the negotiation alter the communication outcome in this scenario?

_____

_____

_____

_____

6. From Provider A's perspective, would you have handled this situation similarly or differently and why?

_____

_____

_____

7. From Provider B's perspective, would you have handled this situation similarly or differently and why?

_____

_____

_____

Key Points

1. Interpersonal communication and health communication are intimately linked. But often interpersonal communication is as important in peer-to-peer and provider-to-provider interactions as it is in provider–patient discourse. Providers in healthcare settings communicate continuously in small groups, with organizations, as well as in dyads. These multifocal and multitask behaviors require a wide variety of verbal and nonverbal communication skills. Recognizing the value of interpersonal and leadership communication, as well as the importance of negotiation skills, are critical to the provider's effectiveness and achieving his/her desired outcomes.

2. Leadership communication is necessary for provider–provider interactions and assuring that a small group's goals are met. So, whether it is a collection of diverse providers working in a team to positively impact a patient's treatment and prognosis, or two providers working to accomplish a single task—leadership and how it is communicated is vital to goal attainment. However, when each provider has a leadership role, sometimes conflicts can occur in trying to reach a consensus, even if both are recommending what each perceives to be in the best interest of the patient.

3. Changing settings for conversations, like moving from the bedside to a private area for a debate or discussion, helps to diffuse some of the potential power issues and reduces the anxiety for those who are not involved. The context for a communication often has a direct affect on the interaction, the interactants, and the outcome. So, be sure to assess the setting in your critical analysis of the communication.

4. Negotiation between individuals of different rank or status can often be enhanced by a mediator or bipartisan third-party. Frequently, such an inclusion can decrease any personal issues between the two negotiators and add some new insight into the proceedings and discussion.

PATIENT COMMUNICATION

WHAT'S WRONG
WITH ME?
10

Before reading the interaction below, please consider the following topics:

Noise in communication channels
- Communication occurs via different channels
  - Air waves (speech)
  - Telephone
  - Electronic (instant messaging or e-mail)
  - Visual (nonverbal cues)
- Noise can occur in any channel
  - A door slamming
  - Someone walking out of a room while a person is talking
  - Intrapersonal communication about a subject other than the one the sender is discussing
  - A television playing while two people are talking
- Unexpected or "bad" news can cause noise in a conversation between a provider and patient
- Noise in a communication channel can make effective communication difficult, if not impossible

Anxious patients
- Anxiety can cause noise in a conversation
  - Patients who are anxious often are preoccupied and have difficulty listening to or assimilating information
- Providers need to try and minimize all noise in communication channels to enhance communication effectiveness and information-sharing

INITIAL INTERACTION

Role play and/or analyze the following example:

John Henderson is a 47-year-old African-American male, who is pacing back and forth across the examination room floor as he waits for the provider. The door opens and Mr. Henderson stops moving and faces the doorway.

Mr. Henderson:	"I'm really not feeling well."
Provider:	"Okay, why don't you sit down? What's bothering you?"
Mr. Henderson:	"Well, I started feeling bad about a week ago and I just keep feeling worse and worse."
Provider:	"I understand, but can you tell me where you feel bad?"
Mr. Henderson:	"I started getting dizzy about a week ago and I thought it would get better, but it hasn't, and now every time I move my head, everything starts spinning. I feel like I want to throw up."
Provider:	"So when aren't you dizzy?"
Mr. Henderson:	"Pretty much all the time, but when I get into bed, if I don't move, that's about the only time. What's wrong with me?"
Provider:	"We need to do some more tests and I need to examine you, but it sounds like you might have labyrinthitis."

Discussion Questions

1. How would you analyze this discussion?

   _____

   _____

   _____

2. Do you agree with the provider's assessment? If so, why? If not, why not?

   _____

   _____

   _____

3. In what way(s) did the patient control the conversation?

   _____

   _____

   _____

4. How did the patient's verbal and nonverbal communication impact the information exchange in this interaction?

_____

_____

_____

_____

5. In what way do you think the patient's aggressive communication style contributed to the abbreviated interaction?

_____

_____

_____

Interactive Activity

- Rewrite (individually or in a group) the interaction between the provider and the patient.
- How would you have handled this patient's behavior and interview differently?
- Compare your rewrite to the Alternate Interaction that follows.

Interaction Rewrite

_____

_____

_____

_____

_____

_____

_____

_____

_____

_____

_____

_____

_____

_____

_____

ALTERNATE INTERACTION

Mr. Henderson was pacing the examination room floor as the provider knocked on the door and enters. The provider walked over to Mr. Henderson, shook his hand, and sat down in a chair.

Provider:	"Hi. Would you like to sit down?"
Mr. Henderson:	"I don't know; I'm not feeling good and I just want to get to feeling better."
Provider:	"I can see that you're concerned and worried, so why don't you tell me what's been going on?"
Mr. Henderson:	"Well, I started feeling bad about a week ago and I just keep feeling worse and worse."
Provider:	"I'm sorry; but the more you can tell me about what's happening, the better it will be."
Mr. Henderson:	"I started getting dizzy about a week ago and I thought it would get better, but it hasn't, and now every time I move my head, everything starts spinning. I feel like I want to throw up."
Provider:	"That's helpful information. What else can you tell me?"
Mr. Henderson:	"I don't know; I've been tired a lot, but that's been going on a while—it's probably related to all the stress at work. But when I got dizzy, I really got worried, 'cause I haven't had a temperature or a cold. I've noticed that I seem to be thirsty a lot and then, because I'm drinking more, I end up peeing a lot. My dad died of cancer, so I'm a little worried about that. Do you have any idea what's wrong with me?"
Provider:	"I think you've provided some great information, and I have some ideas about what might be causing your problems. I don't think it's cancer, but we'll do some tests to rule that out. But let's not get ahead of ourselves. I'd like to get more information. Do you mind if I ask you a number of questions?"
Mr. Henderson:	"If you can figure out why I feel so bad, I'll answer your questions."
Provider:	"Tell me a bit more about your dizziness."
Mr. Henderson:	"Well, it comes and goes; it might be worse when I get up in the morning, but it happens other times too."
Provider:	"Does it only happen when you move your head?"
Mr. Henderson:	"No, it happens sometimes when I'm sitting still."
Provider:	"Okay, now let's talk about your past medical history—any serious illnesses or overnight stays in the hospital?"

Mr. Henderson:	"Nope, no serious illnesses. I had a hernia surgery, but nothing else."
Provider:	"Okay, how about your family history—does anyone in your immediate family have cancer besides your dad?"
Mr. Henderson:	"No, just him and an aunt who had breast cancer."
Provider:	"How about heart attacks or high blood pressure?"
Mr. Henderson:	"My mom has high blood pressure, and my brothers both have high blood pressure, and my grandparents—all of them died of heart attacks."
Provider:	"How about diabetes?"
Mr. Henderson:	"Yeah, we've got a lot of that. I think both my granddads had it; so did a couple of uncles, and I think my mom just started taking pills for it."
Provider:	"Do you drink beer, wine, or liquor?"
Mr. Henderson:	"I have an occasional beer, but I haven't felt like drinking for the last couple of weeks."
Provider:	"Do you smoke cigarettes or have you smoked?"
Mr. Henderson:	"I smoked a little when I was a teenager, but only a few cigarettes a day and only for a couple of years. I didn't like paying all that money for them."
Provider:	"Are you in a committed relationship?"
Mr. Henderson:	"I guess so; we've been married for 15 years."
Provider:	"Have you had any sexually transmitted diseases?"
Mr. Henderson:	"God no!"
Provider:	"Well, I think that's all the questions for now. Let me tell you what I heard you say, and please make sure I got it right. You have been sick for more than a week. It began with a tired-feeling, and then you started getting dizzy. The dizziness comes and goes; it's sometimes worse in the morning, but it doesn't just happen when you move your head. You've been thirsty and eating more lately, and you've been urinating more too. You haven't had any serious illnesses; only one surgery for a hernia, and you don't have a history of sexually transmitted diseases. Your father died of cancer, your mom and brothers have high blood pressure, both your grandfathers had diabetes, and you mom was recently diagnosed with it too. So you have a strong family history for diabetes and heart disease, and your father died of cancer. Did I miss anything?"
Mr. Henderson:	"No, it sounds right. So when are you going to have some answers?"
Provider:	"Good question. We're going to do your examination next, and then we'll get some blood tests and an EKG. I need to have all the results, but here's what I know at this point. Your blood pressure here was normal, so it's unlikely that you have high blood pressure. But I want to check your blood sugar, as well as some other blood levels: cholesterol, liver, kidney tests, etc.

> But I think with your family history of diabetes, that's certainly something
> we have to consider. I just need you to try and be a little patient; we should
> have all the results back by late tomorrow or early Thursday, so we can sit
> down and talk then and I'll be able to answer your questions more fully.
> And I don't want you to think you have a problem if you don't."

Follow-up Discussion

1. How would you compare this interaction with the previous one?

    _____

    _____

    _____

2. How does the provider's interpersonal communication in the alternate scenario
    impact the information exchange?

    _____

    _____

    _____

3. How does the provider's verbal recognition of the patient's anxious behavior impact
    the communication exchange?

    _____

    _____

    _____

4. How does the provider's communication, verbal and nonverbal, serve to decrease
    the patient's anxiety in the second scenario versus the first?

    _____

    _____

    _____

5. Do you think it's a good idea for the provider to discuss his/her preliminary thoughts
    about the patient's symptoms before all the data are available?

    _____

    _____

    _____

6. The provider's initial assessment of the etiology of the patient's symptoms changed from the first to the second interaction. How do you explain the differences?

_____

_____

_____

Key Points

1. Anxious patients can make interactions difficult. It's important for the provider to recognize a patient's anxiety and try to deal with it early in the conversation, so that it does not detract from the exchange of information.

2. In order for patients to listen effectively, they need to have as little "noise" as possible interfering with their active listening. Anxiety can interfere with a patient's ability to listen and provide information and appropriate feedback.

3. Allowing a patient to relate his/her narrative can help decrease anxiety by permitting the patient to communicate his/her concerns and not have the story interrupted with questions.

4. Communicating a provider's thinking, especially for an anxious patient, can help to decrease the patient's concern and increase her/his ability to exchange information and make decisions.

I Understand

11

Before reading the interaction below, please consider the following topics:

Health literacy
- Goes beyond reading ability to comprehension of health communication, both verbal and written
  - Critical to patients' and family members' understanding of providers' messages
- Without appropriate levels of communication, patients' abilities to be properly informed and empowered cannot be assured, and their decision-making capabilities must be questioned

Miscommunication
- Health communication provides countless opportunities for miscommunication, including
  - Health literacy issues
  - Rebellion against authoritarian rule
  - Anxiety or emotional impact of the situation
  - Use of medical or technical jargon
- Lack of feedback
  - To minimize miscommunication, providers need to
    - Restate what they heard the patient say
    - Ask patients to restate what they heard the provider say
    - Observe patients for nonverbal behaviors that indicate confusion or miscommunication

INITIAL INTERACTION

Role play and/or analyze the following example:

Mimi Rosen is a 60-year-old female, who was recently started on blood pressure medication and is back for a follow-up visit. She is sitting on an examination table in a gown when the provider enters the room

Provider:	"Hello, Ms. Rosen. How are you today?"
Ms. Rosen:	"I'm fine. How's my pressure?"
Provider:	"It's still high; did you get the prescriptions filled that I gave you?"
Ms. Rosen:	"Yup."
Provider:	"Are you taking them every day?"
Ms. Rosen:	"Yup."
Provider:	"Well then, we should increase the dosage and have you back in two weeks to check it."
Ms. Rosen:	"Okay."
Provider:	"So, you should double the dose, and I'll see you in two weeks."
Ms. Rosen:	"Okay."
Provider:	"You know hypertension is a very serious disease. It can occlude your blood vessels and lead to a heart attack or stroke."
Ms. Rosen:	"Uh huh."
Provider:	"So, it's important that we get your pressure down and keep it down."
Ms. Rosen:	"Okay."
Provider:	"Are you taking the statin and the baby aspirin we talked about."
Ms. Rosen:	"Sure."

Discussion Questions

1. How would you evaluate the communication in this follow-up visit?

   _____

   _____

   _____

   _____

2. What problems can you identify in the interaction?

_____

_____

_____

_____

3. How would you assess the patient's very brief responses?

_____

_____

_____

_____

4. What other information do you think might have been helpful in determining the possible reasons for the patient's persistently high blood pressure?

_____

_____

_____

_____

5. How does health literacy potentially affect the information-sharing and outcome of this communication?

_____

_____

_____

_____

6. What nonverbal communication behavior(s) do you think might have helped enhance the patient's understanding of her condition and its treatment?

_____

_____

_____

_____

7. What would you have done differently to enhance the provider's communication effectiveness in this scenario?

_____

_____

_____

_____

Interactive Activity

- Rewrite (individually or in a group) the interaction between the provider and the patient.
- How would you alter this interaction to improve the communication effectiveness and patient understanding?
- Compare your rewrite to the Alternate Interaction that follows.

Interaction Rewrite

_____

_____

_____

_____

_____

_____

_____

_____

_____

_____

_____

_____

_____

_____

_____

_____

_____

_____

_____

_____

_____

_____

ALTERNATE INTERACTION

Provider:	"Hi, Ms. Rosen. How are you today?"
Ms. Rosen:	"I'm okay."
Provider:	"I'm glad; but your blood pressure is still up. Do you have any idea why that might be?"
Ms. Rosen:	"You're the doctor; I just come here because they won't feed me at the Community Center if I don't come here."
Provider:	"I'm sorry. Tell me something: are you taking those medicines I gave you prescriptions for last time?"
Ms. Rosen:	"Yup."
Provider:	"Can you tell which ones you take in the morning?"
Ms. Rosen:	"I take a white one, a yellow one, and a pink one."
Provider:	"Good, now what about the evening?"
Ms. Rosen:	"I take the pink one."
Provider:	"Okay, that's the problem. The pink one is the cholesterol pill. You just take it once a day and, instead, you should take the white pill in the evening."
Ms. Rosen:	"Oh, I was wondering why there were more of them than the other ones."
Provider:	"Do you have trouble reading?"
Ms. Rosen:	"I'm not stupid, but big words are tough; and I broke my glasses, so everything's blurry."
Provider:	"Did you talk to anyone about your glasses?"
Ms. Rosen:	"I told Marjorie at the Center."
Provider:	"Is Marjorie a nurse or a social worker?"
Ms. Rosen:	"No, she's my friend."
Provider:	"And you don't have any relatives we can call?"
Ms. Rosen:	"Nope, they're all dead."
Provider:	"I know you eat lunch at the Center; what do you do for breakfast and dinner?"
Ms. Rosen:	"I get a donut for breakfast—I buy a box at the store, with the sugar on them, and then I have a hot dog or lunch meat for dinner."
Provider:	"I'm worried that you're not eating very well and that may be a reason why your cholesterol and your blood pressure are high. I'm going to see if we can get you to an eye doctor, and get you some help from meals-on-wheels. Do you remember that we said last time that salt is not good for people with high blood pressure?"

Ms. Rosen: "I remember, and I told Marjorie that too."

Provider: "Good, so stay away from the salt, and let me try to get my staff to set up the meals-on-wheels and get you an eye appointment."

Ms. Rosen: "Okay, but I need to get back to the Center for lunch."

Provider: "We'll be fast."

Follow-up Discussion

1. What are some of the key differences between the two scenarios?

   _____

   _____

   _____

   _____

2. How does health literacy impact the diagnosis and treatment of this patient?

   _____

   _____

   _____

   _____

3. How is nutrition affecting this patient's care?

   _____

   _____

   _____

   _____

4. Identify the various communication issues that contributed to the patient's treatment problems.

   _____

   _____

   _____

   _____

5. Why did the provider in the initial conversation not identify the possible causes for the patient's persistent hypertension?

_____

_____

_____

_____

6. How did the provider's verbal communication skills, listening, and feedback in the second scenario enhance the information-sharing?

_____

_____

_____

_____

7. How do you assess a person's health literacy and adapt your language choices appropriately?

_____

_____

_____

_____

Key Points

1. Health literacy is a major issue in health communication. Too often providers fail to assess the health literacy level of patients and their families. Consequently, information-exchange and decision-making can be compromised. The use of feedback and questioning can help providers determine the health literacy of patients and their families or care givers.

2. Many times patients want to answer positively to providers' questions about compliance. However, because a patient is taking his/her medication does not mean it is being taken correctly. Providers need to inquire about the way a patient is taking his/her medicine, especially when there are problems. In addition, patients may have other problems contributing to issues with their treatment plan (like paying for prescriptions versus food, or vision problems, etc.). Trying to determine if there are other reasons for a patient's chronic problem can reduce patient–provider interaction time, rather than increase it.

3. The patient's family status, activities of daily living, and nutrition are all important considerations in patient's treatment plans—especially for older patients and those with diminished mental capacities. Providers need to address a patient's lifestyle issues (like economic status and nutrition), and assess their potential impact on the patient's diagnosis and treatment plans.

IT'S BEEN TWO HOURS

12

Before reading the interaction below, please consider the following topics:

Humor
- Commonly used in interpersonal communication
  - To reduce tension or anxiety
  - To humanize the provider
  - To minimize the power inequality in the provider–patient relationship
- Sometimes used by patients to avoid sensitive or upsetting topics
- When used appropriately, can help enhance an interpersonal relationship between the patient and the provider

Communication context
- Communication is context-bound
  - Providers need to communicate differently in a crisis than in an everyday conversation
- Providers need to recognize the impact of context on patient communication and behaviors
  - Because of the context (healthcare), patients are expected to
    - Expose themselves to relative strangers
    - Self-disclose emotionally charged and very personal information to someone who will not reciprocate
    - Accept the provider's role and authority

INITIAL INTERACTION

Role play and/or analyze the following example:

Peter Samuelson is a 62-year-old male, who is sitting in the waiting room of a Fast Track (FT) section of a busy Emergency Department. There are a number of other people in the room as well. Mr. Samuelson is bleeding from a laceration on his forehead. The provider enters the waiting room doorway and shouts.

Provider:	"Mr. Samuelson?"
Mr. Samuelson:	"It's about time. Are you supposed to shout my name like that?"
Provider:	"Hi. We're going into room two."
Mr. Samuelson:	"How come it took you two hours to get to me? I'm bleeding."
Provider:	"Sorry, but we've got a lot of patients and it's first come, first seen, unless it's a life or death emergency. But now it's your turn and let's get you fixed up."
Mr. Samuelson:	"You don't get it. You kept me waiting for two hours and now you act like it's the way it should be handled. What if I was having a heart attack?"
Provider:	"Sir, you're not having heart attack; you've got a small cut on your forehead. Now, I'd like to discuss the problems with healthcare in this country with you, but I've got other patients to see. So, can you tell me how you cut your head?"
Mr. Samuelson:	"Why should I stay here and be treated like this?"
Provider:	"Mr. Samuelson, I'm here to take care of your laceration. So, do you want to tell me how you cut your head, or not?"
Mr. Samuelson:	"Are you deaf, or just dumb? My problem is that I've been waiting and bleeding for two hours, and you come in here and act like this is the way it's supposed to be. I'm your customer!"
Provider:	"Look, you're my patient, not my customer, and I'm not going to be bullied by you. And I don't appreciate you calling me names; so you have two choices—you can sit on the bed and tell me what happened to your head, so I can help you, or you can sign a paper saying you're leaving against medical advice."
Mr. Samuelson:	"No, you're wrong; I have a third choice—I'm leaving; I'm not signing anything. Why would I sign something that relieves you of responsibility when you haven't advised me about a thing? You haven't acknowledged my situation, and all you've done is let me bleed for two hours."

Discussion Questions

1. How would you feel if you had to wait to be seated for two hours at a restaurant, or had to wait in line for two hours at a store?

   _____

   _____

2. Discuss how the context—Emergency Department versus other settings—changes each communicator's perceptions and expectations of the interaction.

   _____

   _____

   _____

3. What role does emotion play in this conversation?

   _____

   _____

   _____

4. How does power impact the interpersonal communication of both interactants?

   _____

   _____

   _____

5. How is power nonverbally communicated in this scenario?

   _____

   _____

   _____

6. In what way is power communicated verbally in this conversation?

   _____

   _____

   _____

7. Does the fact that the patient has a head injury influence how you evaluate this conversation? If so, why? If not, why not?

   _____

   _____

   _____

Interactive Activity

- Rewrite (individually or in a group) the interaction between the provider and the patient.
- How would you alter the outcome of this scenario in terms of changing the patient's perceptions of the provider and the hospital?
- Compare your rewrite to the Alternate Interaction that follows.

Interaction Rewrite

_____

_____

_____

_____

_____

_____

_____

_____

_____

_____

_____

_____

_____

_____

_____

_____

_____

_____

_____

_____

_____

_____

_____

_____

_____

_____

ALTERNATE INTERACTION

Insert your name and/or profession in the appropriate blanks below.

The provider enters the waiting room and goes over and shakes the patient's hand.

Provider: "Hello, Mr. Samuelson? I'm _____, your _____, and I really apologize for your wait. We try very hard to minimize the waiting time, but today we've had two car wrecks and a couple of heart attacks. I know that doesn't make your wait any less, but I did want you to know that we hadn't forgotten about you."

Mr. Samuelson: "Hi. I was getting ready to leave. I'm bleeding here and no one cares."

Provider: "I care! And again, I am sorry that you've had to sit here. But why don't we go back to a room now, and I'll get you examined and get you out of here."

Mr. Samuelson: "I'm not a happy customer. I wouldn't put up with this from any other company."

Provider: "You know, I agree with you. And I know that you are a customer as well as a patient. So I'd like to get you into a room, and then we can talk about your injury and examine your wound."

Mr. Samuelson: "All right. I guess if I went some place else I'd just have to start waiting all over again."

Provider: "Well, that's not the reason I hoped for, but at least you're staying with us and I'll get to treat your cut."

Mr. Samuelson: "This is good; I've made it to a room."

Provider: "Yes, it's progress all right. So now can you please tell me how you cut your forehead?"

Mr. Samuelson: "Well, I don't really know; that's what I was trying to tell the person at the desk. I remember sitting on the toilet, and the next thing I remember is being on the bathroom floor and I was bleeding."

Provider: "I'm surprised they didn't put you in the Emergency Department."

Mr. Samuelson: "They asked me if I was knocked out. I told 'em—no. Nobody knocked me out. I don't know what happened."

Provider: "Okay. So, can you tell me who the President is?"

Mr. Samuelson: "Clinton."

Provider: "And where are we now?"

Mr. Samuelson: "This is a hospital Emergency Room."

Provider: "What day of the week is it?"

Mr. Samuelson: "It's Saturday, January 12, 2008. What's with all the questions?"

Provider: "You're right, I should explain. It sounds like something happened while you were on the toilet. Sometimes if you strain too hard, the blood going to the brain gets stopped for a little bit with the straining and the brain shuts down, like when you turn off a light switch. When that happened, you fell off the toilet and hit your head on the floor. I asked those questions to see if you were still able to think and respond okay to questions about time, place, and person. If you had a brain injury, either before the fall or after it, you might have trouble answering the questions."

Mr. Samuelson: "So are you going to sew this up, or what?"

Provider: "Well, because you blacked out and hit your head, we really need to do a CT scan to make sure you didn't have a bleed inside your brain, or a stroke. And I should check some blood tests to make sure there isn't a different reason why you blacked out. Now, I know you've been waiting a long time, so here's what I'd like to do. I need to finish your examination and order the CT scan. While they're getting ready for your scan, I'll finish my examination, we'll take some blood, and I can sew up your cut and, hopefully, they'll be ready for you then. It will take only 15 minutes or so for the scan and then you can come back, get a bandage and, by then, I should have the reports back from the X-ray doctor and from the lab. Is that okay?"

Mr. Samuelson: "I really don't want to spend any more time here today."

Provider: "I completely understand, but let me explain—you really would want to know if you had a bleed in your head. Now, I don't think you had one, but there's no way to know for sure without the CT scan. And we really should make sure that you're not anemic, or have a low blood sugar, or an electrolyte imbalance."

Mr. Samuelson: "But I thought you said I strained too hard?"

Provider: "You've been listening, that's great. But what I meant to say is that it's possible, even probable that straining caused the fall, but there are other possibilities like a small stroke, or being anemic, or having a low blood sugar, that might have caused it. However, I'm more concerned about what might have happened when you hit your head on the floor. If you hit hard enough to cut your head, you might have caused a bleed inside your skull too. So to be safe, I think you should stay an extra 15 minutes and get the scan."

Mr. Samuelson: "You should be in sales. I do have a headache, so I guess it won't hurt to stay a little longer and get the scan."

Provider: "There's a lot of selling in healthcare, so I'll take that as a compliment. Now I'm going to go order the scan and blood work, plus I'll order you some Ibuprofen for that headache, then I'll come back and finish your examination and sew up your cut."

Mr. Samuelson: "I'll be here."

Provider:	"Just a couple more questions: have you vomited any blood or had blood in your stools?"
Mr. Samuelson:	"Nope."
Provider:	"Any pain when you pee or blood in your urine?"
Mr. Samuelson:	"No."
Provider:	"Okay then, one last question for now: do you have any allergies?"
Mr. Samuelson:	"Just to this place."

Follow-up Discussion

1. What are some of the key differences between the two scenarios?

   _____

   _____

   _____

2. How does the provider's interpersonal communication in the alternate scenario impact the information exchange?

   _____

   _____

   _____

3. In what way does power shift in the second scenario from the first?

   _____

   _____

   _____

4. What nonverbal communication behaviors do you think impacted the patient's perception of the provider?

   _____

   _____

   _____

5. How much does the emotion of the situation contribute to the communication problems and/or solutions?

   _____

   _____

   _____

6. How did the provider's use of explanation and information-sharing impact the patient's decision-making?

_____

_____

_____

7. Would you have handled the conversation from the provider's perspective similarly, or differently, and why?

_____

_____

_____

8. What role did humor play in this conversation?

_____

_____

_____

Key Points

1. Health communication, by its very nature, is often emotionally-charged. In such situations, information-sharing can be lessened, because of the emotional state of the patient and/or family member. Using empathic listening and communicating an awareness of the patient's or family member's situation is a good way to build trust and enhance the interpersonal relationship providers are trying to develop.

2. Power can be a useful tool in communication, but it also can be used in ways that diminish information-sharing and reduce the opportunity for maintaining an interpersonal relationship.

3. Recognizing the patient's situation and acknowledging his/her difficulties are good approaches to building trust and encouraging collaboration.

4. By explaining the reasoning behind ordering tests, or needing extra time, a provider reduces his/her autonomy and treats the patient more as an equal. Therefore, the patient feels less need to rebel against authority, and may find it easier to agree with the proposed course of action. The key is providing more information and fewer commands.

WHY DO I HAVE TO WAIT FOR AN MRI?
13

Before reading the interaction below, please consider the following topics:

Self-disclosure
- Is one of the hallmarks of an evolving interpersonal relationship
- Is critical to effective health communication
  - Requires patients to disclose sensitive and private revelations about themselves
  - In the provider–patient context, does not result in provider reciprocating as in most interpersonal relationships

Patient empowerment
- Patients need knowledge about their health and treatment options to make well-informed decisions
- Health information can come from a wide variety of sources, some credible and some not as credible
- Empowerment allows patients to have influence in their own healthcare decision-making
- Providers can help patients by providing information, encouraging feedback and questions, and collaborating with patients in the decision-making process

INITIAL INTERACTION

Role play and/or analyze the following example:

Sarah Aronson stood in the waiting room and talked through the receptionist window to the person on the other side. Ms. Aronson is a 33-year-old woman, who has a history of recurring headaches. She was told by her provider that she needed an MRI, and she has returned because she hasn't been able to schedule the test for nearly a week.

Receptionist: "Ms. Aronson, I'm getting someone to speak with you."

(The provider enters the receptionist's office and begins talking to the patient through the window.)

Provider: "Ms. Aronson, is there a problem?"

Ms. Aronson: "Why do I have to wait for an MRI?"

Provider: "I'm not sure. Let me see what I can find out."

(The provider closes the glass window separating the receptionist's office from the waiting room and turns toward the receptionist.)

Provider: "Do you know what the problem is?"

Receptionist: "I could have told her if she'd asked me—her insurance wanted a letter from you, so I faxed that to them yesterday. It's all about them approving it. Then I can schedule it."

Provider: "You couldn't have told her that?"

Receptionist: "I did tell her that, but she still insisted on talking to you."

(The provider turns back to the window and slides the glass window open.)

Provider: "Ms. Aronson, we have sent your insurance company the information they requested, so I'm guessing they'll be calling today or tomorrow with the authorization."

Ms. Aronson: "My head still hurts, and I can't believe it takes a week to get the MRI. Is there anything else you can do?"

Provider: "I've done all I can do. Now we just have to wait until we hear back from them. I'll see you for your appointment next week and, hopefully by then, the MRI will be done."

Ms. Aronson: "My head's killing me, and you're hopeful."

(The provider closed the sliding glass window.)

Discussion Questions

1. What are the major issues you have with the communication in this interaction?

   _____

   _____

   _____

   _____

2. If you were the patient, what are the problems you would have with the communication?

   _____

   _____

   _____

   _____

3. How does the setting (waiting room–receptionist's office) impact the communication in this scenario?

   _____

   _____

   _____

4. How does the provider's loss of autonomy in ordering treatments potentially affect his/her communication?

   _____

   _____

   _____

5. Is there a Health Insurance Portability and Accountability Act (HIPAA) issue involved in this interaction? If so, what is it and why?

   _____

   _____

   _____

6. How would you have handled this situation differently? Be specific.

   _____

   _____

   _____

Interactive Activity

- Rewrite (individually or in a group) the interaction between the provider and the patient.
- Try to find a way that enhances the relationship between the provider and patient.
- Compare your rewrite to the Alternate Interaction that follows.

Interaction Rewrite

_____

_____

_____

_____

_____

_____

_____

_____

_____

_____

_____

_____

_____

_____

_____

_____

_____

_____

_____

_____

_____

_____

_____

_____

_____

_____

_____

_____

_____

_____

_____

_____

ALTERNATE INTERACTION

The provider enters the receptionist's office as the receptionist and Ms. Aronson are having a conversation through the sliding glass window that separates the office from the waiting room.

Provider:	"What's the problem? Hi, Ms. Aronson!"
Receptionist:	"She's upset about not getting her MRI, but I faxed the letter you wrote to the case manager yesterday."
Ms. Aronson:	"I don't understand why I can't get my MRI."
Provider:	"Let's not discuss this here. Why don't you come back to my office?" (They go to the provider's office.)
Provider:	"I understand that it's frustrating not getting the MRI, but the insurance company has to preapprove all nonemergency MRIs. But let's talk about your headache. How is it feeling?"
Ms. Aronson:	"Well, it's a little better with the new medicine, but it's not completely gone. I am just worried that maybe I have a tumor—I saw on the Internet that tumors can cause headaches."

Provider: "So you're worried. I can understand that, but you should know that most headaches are NOT caused by a tumor. As I told you, I'm only doing this to be complete; if I thought it were something serious, I assure you we would have talked about it. You've got an appointment with the neurologist for next month, and we want to make sure we have all the base-line tests done that she'll need when she sees you. So, that's why we did the blood tests and ordered the MRI."

Ms. Aronson: "Okay, but I just read so much stuff on the Internet and it was really scary."

Provider: "I know, and often it's really good to learn everything you can about something, but sometimes, when you're not even sure what you're dealing with, reading too much about problems that you don't even have can increase your stress and anxiety. So, let me ask Mary, the receptionist, to call the case manager while you're here and see if we can get this approved and scheduled. That way we'll be sure it's done before you see Dr. Finegold."

Ms. Aronson: "That would be such a relief. I'm really sorry to bother you, but it would be so great not to have to worry about that."

(The provider picks up the phone and dials.)

Provider: "Mary, can you call Ms. Aronson's case manager and see if you can get her MRI approved? Okay Ms. Aronson, she's going to make the call and she'll let you know what she finds out."

Ms. Aronson: "Thank you so much."

Follow-up Discussion

1.   What are some of the key differences between the two scenarios?

_____

_____

_____

2.   How does the provider's willingness to talk to Ms. Aronson in her/his office impact the conversation?

_____

_____

_____

3.   Is the time required to talk with Ms. Aronson worth the time lost by the provider? If so, why? If not, why not?

_____

_____

_____

4. How do the patient's efforts at self-education and empowerment affect the outcome of the two scenarios?

    _____

    _____

    _____

5. How much does the patient's self-disclosure about the Internet searches alter the outcome between the first and the alternate scenarios?

    _____

    _____

    _____

6. How did the provider–patient relationship evolve in the alternate versus the original scenario? What role did active listening play in this change?

    _____

    _____

    _____

7. How would you have handled the conversation from the provider's perspective: similarly, or differently, and why?

    _____

    _____

    _____

Key Points

1. Communication often gets confused by emotional situations, and health communication is almost always impacted by emotions. So, what may seem on the surface as one issue may very well be only the smoke-screen for the real problem. With the increased availability of information on the Internet, providers need to be aware of the potential risk for misinformation, increased anxiety, and miscommunication.

2. With the increase in insurance company preapprovals for nonemergency diagnostic tests, communication between the provider and patient, or the provider's office and the patient, about expectations is critical.

3. Providers need to be extremely conscious of conversations with patients about their health that occur in public settings. It's important to remember to avoid discussions in public, and to protect the patient's privacy by saving such interactions for behind closed doors.

I'm Feeling Better, But . . .
14

Before reading the interaction below, please consider the following topics:

Gender communication
- Gender and sex are different
- Sex is related to anatomy (penis is male; vagina is female)
- Gender is not related to anatomy, but to certain traits including
  - Masculine gender is aggressive, competitive, independent
  - Feminine gender is collaborative, participatory, docile
- Patients use language based on their gender
  - Masculine-gendered males or females use language to accomplish goals
  - Feminine-gendered males or females use language to build relationships
- Providers need to assess patients' gender and communication styles, and not assume that they are the same for all males or all females
  - Masculine-gendered individuals can be expected to communicate less information
  - Feminine-gendered patients are more likely to want to talk more about their illness or condition and share more information

Miscommunication
- Occurs for a wide variety of reasons including
  - Disparity in health literacy between provider and patient
  - Provider's use of technical or medical jargon
  - Patients limiting their supply of information and/or detail
  - Providers and patients failing to use feedback to assess understanding

INITIAL INTERACTION

Role play and/or analyze the following example.
Insert your name and/or profession in the appropriate blanks below.

Harold Winter, a 44-year-old white male, had been seen two days earlier in the provider's office with a paronychial infection of his right index finger. He was given a prescription for an antibiotic and told to call back if he had any problems. He called the provider's office and left a message for the provider to call him back.

Provider:	Harold, this is _____. I heard you called."
Mr. Winter:	"Hi. You said to call back if I wasn't doing well."
Provider:	"What's going on?"
Mr. Winter:	"Well, I'm taking the antibiotic and I'm feeling better, but now my stomach is bothering me."
Provider:	"Are you taking the Ibuprofen?"
Mr. Winter:	"Yeah, three of them every six hours, just like you said."
Provider:	"Well, I'm guessing it's the Ibuprofen, so why don't you stop taking that and just finish the antibiotic."
Mr. Winter:	"Okay, but my wife thinks I need to go to a hand surgeon."
Provider:	"For what? You bit your nail and got it infected—you don't need a hand surgeon for that kind of an infection."
Mr. Winter:	"I didn't bite my nail; I cut it too close. You don't have to holler at me."
Provider:	"I'm not hollering! I'm just trying to get you to understand that the treatment for your infection wouldn't be any different if you went to a hand surgeon. You need warm soaks and antibiotics. Plus, you need to take Ibuprofen or acetaminophen for pain. Let me know if you have any more problems, but you don't need a hand surgeon."
Mr. Winter:	"Okay, I'll tell my wife. But she's not going to be very happy."
Provider:	"Well, you can tell her you're going to be just fine."
	(Ten minutes later Mrs. Winter calls the office.)
Receptionist:	"Mrs. Winter, under HIPAA, the provider cannot talk to you about your husband's condition."
Mrs. Winter:	"Listen, my husband signed a release for you to talk with me."
Receptionist:	"Oh, all right. I'll have Mr. Winter's provider call you back."
Mrs. Winter:	"I'll wait for an hour, but if I don't get a call back by then, I'm calling our attorney."
Receptionist:	"You're calling a lawyer if you don't get called back in an hour?"

Mrs. Winter: "No, I'm calling a lawyer if I don't talk with someone, because my husband's finger is worse. Plus, I think the antibiotic is giving him diarrhea, and I think he needs a referral to a hand surgeon, and our insurance won't pay without a referral."

Receptionist: "I'll make sure you get a call back shortly."

Discussion Questions

1. What problems did you identify in these two interactions?

_____

_____

_____

_____

2. If you were the patient, how would you feel about the communication you had with the provider?

_____

_____

_____

3. How does the format (a phone call) help or hinder the effective exchange of information between the patient and the provider, and the patient's wife and the receptionist?

_____

_____

_____

_____

4. How does the patient's ability to describe his problem potentially interfere with effective communication?

_____

_____

_____

5. Based on all the communication in this scenario, what do you think is going on?

_____

_____

_____

6. How would you have handled this situation differently? Be specific.

    _____

    _____

    _____

7. What impact on current and future communication do you think Mrs. Winter's threat of talking to an attorney will have?

    _____

    _____

    _____

Interactive Activity

- Rewrite (individually or in a group) the interaction between the provider and the patient.
- Try to find a way to enhance the relationship between the provider and patient, to maximize the exchange of information and minimize everyone's frustration.
- Compare your rewrite to the Alternate Interaction that follows.

Interaction Rewrite

_____

_____

_____

_____

_____

_____

_____

_____

_____

_____

_____

_____

_____

_____

_____

_____

_____

ALTERNATE INTERACTION

Insert your name and/or profession in the appropriate blanks below.

Receptionist: "Hi. I've got Mr. Winter on the phone. Here's his chart; he's got a problem."

Provider: "Hi, Mr. Winter. It's _____. How's your finger doing?"

Mr. Winter: "I'm doing better, but my stomach is bothering me."

Provider: "Tell me what's going on with your stomach?"

Mr. Winter: "It hurts and I've got diarrhea."

Provider: "Well, that's not good. Are your stools loose, or are you having lots of bowel movements?"

Mr. Winter: "Both I guess; my stools are loose and I've gone about five or six times since midnight. And I'm cramping."

Provider: "I'm sorry. Sometimes the Ibuprofen can cause you to have stomach pain, and sometimes the antibiotic can cause stomach upset and diarrhea, so I'm guessing we need to stop the combination penicillin and sulfa prescription and start a different one."

Mr. Winter: "Okay, that sounds good. But my wife thinks I need to see a hand surgeon."

Provider: "Well, we can do that, but I should see you first. Can you come in this afternoon around 4 P.M.?"

Mr. Winter: "Sure."

Provider: "Great; and please bring your wife, so we can all talk and make sure I get everyone's questions answered. But no more of the antibiotic and let's hold off on the Ibuprofen as well. If it's hurting a lot, then take some acetaminophen, okay?"

Mr. Winter: "Got it. We'll see you at four."

(Mr. and Mrs. Winter are waiting in an examination room when the provider knocks and then enters.)

Provider: "Hi, Mr. and Mrs. Winter. I'm sorry you had to come in, but I think I need to look at that finger, and talk with you about what's been going on since you were here last."

Mr. Winter: "Thanks, I'm sorry we're bothering you."

Mrs. Winter: "I think his finger is worse, and he's not telling you because he's afraid you're going to cut it open."

Provider: "I agree. It does look worse. I'm glad you came in—this needs to be drained and we need to change you to a different antibiotic."

Mrs. Winter: "That's what I thought. Do you think we need to see a hand surgeon?"

Provider: "Well, I can refer him, but I can tell you the hand surgeon would do the same thing I'm going to do. The infection is sealed in that spot right there where it's so swollen and red. It's not in his blood stream; but it's hard for the antibiotics to get to it, so we need to open it and drain it. That's what the hand surgeon would do too."

Mrs. Winter: "Well, if you're sure that's all it needs, then I guess we don't need to go to a surgeon."

Mr. Winter: "Well, I'm glad you think that it's all right, but it's my finger he's talking about cutting on."

Provider: "Mr. Winter, let me explain exactly what's going to happen and then you can make your decision. No matter who you have open this, the procedure will be the same. We need to put a little numbing medicine under the skin, like what the dentist does for your teeth. It will sting for a minute or two maximum, then it won't hurt anymore for an hour or two. While it's numb, I'll make a small opening in the swollen area and let the pus come out. Then we'll leave it open to drain. It should feel much better after the infection is out of there."

Mr. Winter: "Okay, if that's all you're talking about doing, then I guess I'd like to just get it done."

Provider: "Good, I'm glad you're here and that you are going to let me fix this. Do you have any allergies to medicines?"

Mr. Winter: "No."

Provider: "Okay, so while I'm getting the things I need to do this, let me just go over the instructions. First, I'll give you a new prescription. Second, stop both the antibiotic and the Ibuprofen, and be sure to go on clear liquids only, for 24 hours. If you have any black or bloody bowel movements, give me a call right away or go to the Emergency Department. I would expect the diarrhea and loose stools to return to normal in a couple of days. If they don't, please call me. I'm going to leave the wound open—no sutures and no drain—so you'll just need to wash it with soap and then put on triple-antibiotic ointment and a band-aid, at least once a day. Take the new antibiotic until it's all gone. It shouldn't upset your stomach, but I'm going to take a culture of your wound when I get it opened, and we'll call you if it shows we need to use a different antibiotic."

Mrs. Winter: "So we might have to have a third antibiotic?"

Provider: "I don't think so, but to be safe, we'll do a culture and that will tell us which antibiotics are best against the infection you've got. If we need to, we'll change, but I doubt that will be necessary."

Follow-up Discussion

1. What are some of the key differences between the two scenarios for the provider, patient, and spouse?

   _____

   _____

   _____

   _____

   _____

2. What difference do you think it made to have the patient come into the office versus just having a discussion on the phone?

   _____

   _____

   _____

3. Do you think most providers would have asked the patient and his wife to come in to be examined? If so, why? If not, why not?

   _____

   _____

   _____

4. What role does the sex of the patient play in the miscommunication in the first scenario?

   _____

   _____

   _____

5. How does the provider–patient communication change when a patient brings a family member with him/her into the examination room, and the spouse/family member asks questions, etc.? Do you encourage or discourage the practice and why?

   _____

   _____

   _____

   _____

6. How did the provider's communication in the alternate scenario decrease the need for a referral? Be specific.

_____

_____

_____

7. Why not just refer the patient and let the hand surgeon deal with the wife and the patient's problems?

_____

_____

_____

■Key Points

1. Masculine-gendered individuals tend to be more independent and less inquisitive about their care and treatment. Feminine-gendered patients frequently want to participate more in their care, discuss their problems and treatment options, and ask questions. For providers trying to understand the gendered communication of their patients, it is helpful to recognize who needs more information and who needs more probing for details.

2. While appropriate referrals to specialists are a key to effective healthcare delivery, referring just to avoid extended communication, or to minimize conflicts, should not be a standard of practice. Providers need to understand fully the patient's complaint, and to assess the medical need for referral versus the need to communicate more effectively with a patient and his/her family members.

3. Providers need to constantly be aware of the potential communication problems related to telephone consultations. Even the most simple questions and answers can create dilemmas related to the lack of nonverbal feedback and the lack of objective data from visibly examining the patient. In spite of the time issues caused by seeing patients versus talking to them on the phone, providers must carefully weigh the benefits versus the risk in terms of non-face-to-face interactions and assessments.

WE DON'T KNOW WHAT TO DO

15

Before reading the interaction below, please consider the following topics:

Geriatric communication
- Older adults are more likely to communicate differently than younger adults; specifically older patients typically
  - Ask fewer questions of providers
  - Assert themselves less
- Providers may interpret the older patient's silence or lack of questions as disinterest or being well-informed
- May require more time than providers expect to spend talking with patients

Noise in the communication channel
- Elderly patients frequently bring a caregiver or family member with them to the interaction with a provider
  - Providers need to recognize the role of the caregiver or family member, and try to minimize any confusion related to the additional communicator's questions or responses
- While it's important to communicate with the caregiver, it's also important not to ignore the patient in the conversation
- Noise can distract and interfere with effective communication, but a caregiver or family member can often help to decrease the noise and increase the information-sharing, comprehension, and decision-making

INITIAL INTERACTION

Role play and/or analyze the following example:

Julie and John Wilson are married and both in their late 70s. John was just diagnosed with Type II diabetes, and the couple has driven from the provider's office, where they got the news, to their daughter, JoAnn's, home.

Mrs. Wilson: "Hi. We need your help; we don't know what to do."

Mr. Wilson: "They said I've got diabetes, so I'm scared."

JoAnn: "Well, what did they tell you?"

Mrs. Wilson: "That's our problem; we're not really sure. We thought it was just going to be a regular visit, and then the provider started talking about diabetes and how dangerous it was, and how important it is to change what we eat and when we eat, and that we'd need to do finger sticks. It was just too much."

JoAnn: "Okay, I'm sure it was too much, but what did they tell you to do first?"

Mr. Wilson: "I'm supposed to see someone who will teach us about diabetes and what to do."

JoAnn: "Great, so we can all go with you and help figure this out. Did you get a prescription?"

Mr. Wilson: "Yes, but they said not to get it filled till after we meet with the diabetes person."

Mrs. Wilson: "We just didn't know what to do until then."

JoAnn: "Did they set up a meeting for you?"

Mr. Wilson: "I don't know."

JoAnn: "Okay, then let's call the office and see if we can get some answers."
(JoAnn calls the provider's office.)

JoAnn: "Hi. This is Mr. Wilson's daughter. He was just there and still has some questions; can we talk with the provider?"

Receptionist: "I can take a phone number and have her call you back, but because of HIPAA rules, she'll need to talk to your dad or mom."

JoAnn: "Well, she talked to them and they're confused, so I was trying to help. I didn't want to schedule another appointment."

Receptionist: "Do you have a speaker phone?"

JoAnn: "Yeah, I think so."

Receptionist: "Okay. Then the provider can call your father on that number and if your dad says it's okay, you can be on the speaker phone and hear what is said and ask questions. We just need your dad's permission for you to be included."

Discussion Questions

1. What are a few of the communication problems raised in this scenario?

   _____

   _____

   _____

   _____

2. How do you think the patient's diagnosis impacted the communication?

   _____

   _____

   _____

3. How did the patient's and his wife's ages affect the communication with the provider?

   _____

   _____

   _____

4. In what ways has HIPAA made communication more challenging for providers, patients, and family members?

   _____

   _____

   _____

5. Do you think the provider could have anticipated these communication problems? If so, why? If not, why not?

   _____

   _____

   _____

   _____

6. How would you have handled this situation differently? Be specific.

   _____

   _____

   _____

   _____

Interactive Activity

- Rewrite (individually or in a group) the interaction between the provider, patient, and family members.
- Try to find a way to minimize the confusion and improve the communication in the scenario.
- Compare your rewrite to the Alternate Interaction that follows.

Interaction Rewrite

_____

_____

_____

_____

_____

_____

_____

_____

_____

_____

_____

_____

_____

_____

_____

_____

_____

_____

_____

_____

_____

_____

_____

_____

_____
_____
_____
_____
_____
_____
_____
_____
_____
_____
_____
_____
_____
_____

ALTERNATE INTERACTION

The provider is meeting with Mr. and Mrs. Wilson and brings them to the office, not an examination room.

Provider: "How are you doing, Mr. Wilson?"

Mr. Wilson: "I'm okay; still peeing a lot."

Provider: "That's why I wanted to talk to you and Mrs. Wilson. Remember we did those blood tests last time you were in? Well the tests show you have diabetes."

Mr. Wilson: "That's not good."

Mrs. Wilson: "Oh my God! Your mother had that."

Provider: "Well, it's not that bad. We just have to get you on a treatment plan and then check you regularly."

Mrs. Wilson: "I can't give shots; I get dizzy just thinking about it."

Provider: "Let's slow down; there are no shots. You'll need to take a pill and we'll get you on a diabetic diet, and a little exercise, and you should do just great."

Mr. Wilson:	"That doesn't sound too bad."
Provider:	"I've got some information for you, so you can read about it. Then we're going to get you in to see our diabetes educator; she's terrific and she'll make sure you understand what you need to do and when. She'll help you with a plan and a calendar, and go over what foods are better to eat and which foods are not as healthy."
Mrs. Wilson:	"I don't know what to do."
Provider:	"I understand, it's a lot of information. That's why we're giving you some things to take home and read, and why you're meeting with me and then with Kim, the diabetes educator. We'll both see you again in a couple of weeks to see how things are going, and you can call Kim or me with any questions."
Mr. Wilson:	"I'll bet our daughter, JoAnn, will have some questions—can she call?"
Provider:	"Of course. I'll get you a form to sign so it's okay for us to talk with her about your health. It's just to protect your confidentiality."
Mr. Wilson:	"Sure, I'll be happy to sign."
Provider:	"Now, I'd like to take just a minute to see what you heard me say today. Can you tell me what we just talked about?"
Mr. Wilson:	"Well, let's see—you said I have diabetes, but not the kind that needs a shot. I need to eat differently and exercise. And we're going to talk with someone else about all this."
Mrs. Wilson:	"And you said that we could call and so could JoAnn."
Provider:	"You two did great! But remember, I've given you information to read and it lists the next steps, and I'm sure JoAnn will want to read it too. And we're going to meet with you again in two weeks to see how things are going. Now before you go meet with Kim, do you have any more questions for me?"

Follow-up Discussion

1. List all the nonverbal behaviors that you think positively impacted the exchange of information in the second scenario?

   _____

   _____

   _____

   _____

   _____

2. What was the provider's purpose in using the office versus an examination room?

_____

_____

_____

_____

3. What are your thoughts about having the diabetes educator scheduled to see the patient and his wife on the same day as they get the diagnosis? What are some of the negative consequences?

_____

_____

_____

_____

4. What role does the age of the patient and his wife play in the communication exchange?

_____

_____

_____

5. How does the media's portrayal of chronic diseases, like diabetes, affect how patients respond to such a diagnosis?

_____

_____

_____

_____

6. What do you think is the value or nonvalue of giving the patient and his wife the handouts and written next steps? Be specific.

_____

_____

_____

_____

7. Why did the provider ask Mr. and Mrs. Wilson what they had heard her say about the patient's condition?

_____

_____

_____

_____

▌Key Points

1. Older patients often need more time to process information. In addition, the emotionally-charged diagnosis of diabetes, especially for an older couple, should be expected to generate many questions and some difficulty processing the information. To help minimize this and decrease the time needed to communicate effectively, providers need to develop some communication strategies to deal with the situation prior to the interaction.

2. Trying to find ways to minimize noise in the communication channel is very important to effective information-sharing. Noise can come from many things, not the least of which can be internal from emotional responses to troubling news, like a diagnosis of a chronic disease. The more providers can recognize the many potential causes of noise in a communication channel, the easier it will be for patients and providers to interact effectively. One way to minimize noise is to provide a setting that is relaxed and comfortable. Another is to provide handouts that can be used to reinforce what was said.

3. Feedback is very important to interpersonal communication, and feedback comes from nonverbal cues, like head nodding, or eye movements. But it can also come from verbal behaviors like asking a patient and/or family members to state what was heard, so the provider can assess if there was any miscommunication. It's important to always remember that listening is different from hearing. A person can have the anatomic and physiologic capabilities to hear, but listening requires effort and focus on the receiver's part. Feedback is one way to assess listening and to alter any misperceptions or misunderstandings.

I HURT MY BACK

16

Before reading the interaction below, please consider the following topics:

Stereotyping
- Occurs when a person gets classified because of a perception about his/her group membership. For example
  - All older patients may be perceived as not being sexually active
  - All good students are not risk takers
- Providers differentiate themselves from their patients when they stereotype
- Stereotyping can cause providers to miscommunicate or even mis-diagnose because of misperceptions

Verbal aggression
- Aggressiveness and argumentativeness are not the same
- Verbal aggression occurs when speakers attack others personally, instead of the other person's ideas
- When one person uses verbal aggression, it is not unusual for the other communicator to become defensive and respond in kind
- Verbal aggression does not lead to effective communication

INITIAL INTERACTION

Role play and/or analyze the following example:

Sara Dominick is a 19-year-old woman in the Emergency Department (ED) for low back pain. She has multiple piercings of the eyebrows, nose, lip, tongue, and ears. She also has tattoos on her neck, arms, and legs. The provider on duty pulls back the curtain separating the cubicle from the rest of the ED. Ms. Dominick is sitting on the gurney, crying.

Provider:	"Why are you crying?"
Ms. Dominick:	"I'm in pain! I've been waiting for hours."
Provider:	"Okay, so where's your pain?"
Ms. Dominick:	"It's in my back. Can you give me something for it?"
Provider:	"Where in your back?"
Ms. Dominick:	"It's right here, above my butt."
Provider:	"So why don't you stand up and show me how far you can bend over?"
Ms. Dominick:	"If I could bend over, I wouldn't have waited for three hours to see you. I can't bend over."
Provider:	"Without moving your feet, turn as far as you can to your left. Now turn to the right. Okay, now lay down on your back."
Ms. Dominick:	"Do you understand it hurts to move? Why don't you give me some pain medicine before you have me trying to do all this?"
Provider:	"Ms. Dominick, I have to know the cause of your pain before I can give you anything for it. I need to make sure it's not caused by a kidney stone or something internal, and then I'll get you some medicine."
Ms. Dominick:	"It's not a kidney stone; I hurt my back and I came here for medicine to make it better. Are you listening to me?"
Provider:	"I'm listening. It sounds like you want pain medicine and I'm trying to determine what type of pain medicine to give you. But you're not cooperating very much, so it's making the process a lot more difficult and time-consuming."
Ms. Dominick:	"What are you calling me—a drug addict? I'm no junkie, I'm just in pain. What a place! If I hadn't been waiting so long, I would leave."
Provider:	"I'm not calling you anything; I'm just trying to help you, but if you want to go somewhere else, you can sign out against medical advice."
Ms. Dominick:	"You're an asshole!"
Provider:	"Well, I'm the asshole who can write prescriptions, so you choose—work with me, or sign out against medical advice?"

Discussion Questions

1. What are a few of the communication problems raised in this scenario?

   _____

   _____

   _____

   _____

2. How do you think the patient's demeanor, tattoos, and piercings impacted the inter-action?

   _____

   _____

   _____

   _____

3. Do you think the patient's request for pain medicine changed the provider's per-ception of the patient's complaints?

   _____

   _____

   _____

4. How do preconceptions and stereotypes about drug-seekers and drug-seeking behav-iors affect interpersonal communication and interpersonal relationship-development in settings like the Emergency Department?

   _____

   _____

   _____

   _____

5. How did verbally aggressive behavior (name calling) impact the exchange of information?

   _____

   _____

   _____

   _____

Interactive Activity

- Rewrite (individually or in a group) the interaction between the provider and the patient.
- Try to write a scenario that allows the provider and the patient to effectively share information and meet each person's expectations.
- Compare your rewrite to the Alternate Interaction that follows.

Interaction Rewrite

_____

_____

_____

_____

_____

_____

_____

_____

_____

_____

_____

_____

_____

_____

_____

_____

_____

_____

_____

_____

_____

_____

_____

_____
_____
_____
_____
_____
_____
_____
_____
_____
_____
_____
_____
_____
_____
_____
_____
_____
_____

ALTERNATE INTERACTION

Insert your name and/or profession in the appropriate blanks below.

Provider:	"Ms. Dominick, hi. My name is _____, and I'm a _____. How are you doing?"
Ms. Dominick:	"I'm in pain—my back is really hurting."
Provider:	"I'm sorry; I'll get you some pain medicine as soon as I've finished my examination."
Ms. Dominick:	"It's really hurting!"
Provider:	"So tell me what happened?"
Ms. Dominick:	"I was helping my mom move and we were lifting boxes all day yesterday, and today I can hardly move it hurts so bad."

Provider:	"That sounds really painful; have you had back problems before?"
Ms. Dominick:	"No, this is my first time."
Provider:	"Do you have any serious past medical problems?"
Ms. Dominick:	"No, I'm just in pain."
Provider:	"How about any problems with numbness or tingling in your arms or legs?"
Ms. Dominick:	"No."
Provider:	"Okay, we're almost done with the questions. Do you take any medicines every day?"
Ms. Dominick:	"Birth control pills, that's it."
Provider:	"Any allergies to medicines?"
Ms. Dominick:	"No."
Provider:	"Any blood in your urine, or pain when you urinate?"
Ms. Dominick:	"No. Can you just get me something for my back?"
Provider:	"I'm going to order you a pain pill, just as soon as I feel your abdomen and check your back."
Ms. Dominick:	"Thank you!"

Follow-up Discussion

1. List all the nonverbal behaviors that you think positively impacted the exchange of information in the second scenario?

    _____

    _____

    _____

    _____

    _____

2. Why do you think the communication did not decline into verbal aggression in the alternate scenario?

    _____

    _____

    _____

    _____

    _____

3. Do you think an interpersonal relationship can be initiated in such a short conversation? If so, why? If not, why not?

    _____

    _____

    _____

4. How does the patient's request for pain medicine impact the provider's assessment and communication?

    _____

    _____

    _____

5. How do you use a patient's communication (verbal and nonverbal cues), including their artifacts (clothing, jewelry, tattoos, etc.), to help in your assessment of drug-seeking behaviors?

    _____

    _____

    _____

6. How did the provider's willingness to acknowledge the patient's pain and discuss his/her plans to medicate affect the interaction? Be specific.

    _____

    _____

    _____

    _____

Key Points

1. Stereotypes are a frequent problem for effective communication. First impressions are all too often clouded by our perceptions of the individual, based on the person's nonverbal communication and our previous experiences. We make determinations about people by stereotyping them, based on their posture, gaze, and kinesics. Just as frequently we allow their artifacts: clothing, tattoos, jewelry, piercings, hair styles, etc. to color our perceptions of the individual. Instead of listening to the person, communicators let nonverbal cues lead to stereotypes that interfere with the message the person is trying to communicate. Healthcare providers need to work diligently to keep stereotypes from influencing their perceptions while, at the same time, using all the data they can gather to enhance their assessments and decision-making. But that requires using both nonverbal and verbal messages in your evaluation.

2. Patients in pain want pain relief, but with drug-seeking patients an issue, especially in Urgent Care and Emergency Departments, it can be difficult to assess who needs pain medicine and who does not. The more a provider can use interpersonal communication to encourage an information-exchange and build an interpersonal relationship, the easier it will be to assess the patient's symptoms and need for pain management.

3. Verbal aggression occurs when one communicator chooses to attack another's personal characteristics or values. Verbal aggression frequently leads to reciprocation and a rapid decline in effective communication. Because of the emotional intensity of health communication, conflicts can arise and providers need to be aware of the risk of verbal aggression. Once a person resorts to verbally aggressive communication, the provider needs to recognize it and not retaliate or reciprocate with verbal aggression toward the patient. Instead, acknowledging the use of verbal aggression via feedback to the communicator, and explaining that it will not be tolerated, is imperative for a successful interpersonal communication exchange.

THE MEDIA AND HEALTH COMMUNICATION

III

ERECTILE DYSFUNCTION

17

Before reading the interaction below, please consider the following topics:

Emotional communication
- Health communication, because of patients' fears and concerns, is impacted by emotions
  - Emotional stress can alter physiologic responses like pulse and blood pressure
  - Emotional conversations can require more time
- Providers need to be aware of their own behaviors, and not keep patients from discussing sensitive or emotional topics

Self-disclosure
- Helps relationships and information-sharing grow
- Generally increases as the relationship between provider and patient increases
- The better the relationship, the more likely people are to disclose negative information about themselves
- In relationships, both communicators tend to be more satisfied when the amount of self-disclosure seems appropriate—not too much or too little

INITIAL INTERACTION

Role play and/or analyze the following example.
Insert your name and/or profession in the appropriate blanks below.

Pietro Santuli is a 60-year-old male with Type II diabetes. He's recently changed providers because his insurance changed and it no longer covered his previous provider of 15 years. He is seeing this provider for the first time. The patient is seated on an examination table, wearing nothing but his underwear and a patient gown. The provider enters the room.

Provider: "Mr. Santuli. Hi, I'm _____, your _____."

Mr. Santuli: "Hi, please call me Pietro."

Provider: "Okay, Peter. What can I do for you today?"

Mr. Santuli: "My insurance company—they tell me I got to see you for my sugar."

Provider: "Okay, I see you're a diabetic. Are you having any problems?"

Mr. Santuli: "Not really; I just had to change doctors and they said to come to you."

Provider: "So you're just here for a sugar test?"

Mr. Santuli: "Sure."

Provider: "I've got your records here from Dr. Lunaci, so it looks like you're doing a good job keeping your blood sugar under control. Any problems with your feet?"

Mr. Santuli: "Nope, they're fine."

Provider: "Good. Any sores that aren't healing?"

Mr. Santuli: "Nope."

Provider: "Any numbness in your hands or feet?"

Mr. Santuli: "No."

Provider: "Any increased thirst? How's your weight?"

Mr. Santuli: "My weight is just about the same as it has been for the past few years."

Provider: "That's good; it's just a bit high, so we'll talk about taking off a few pounds after I finish my examination. So let's get you checked out and that blood drawn, and then we'll talk about some things for you to do."

Mr. Santuli: "Okay, but I'll need a new prescription."

Provider: "No problem; let's just see what the blood tests and my examination show, and we'll get you all fixed up."

Discussion Questions

1. How would you evaluate this communication exchange?

    _____
    _____
    _____
    _____

2. Do you think the provider established an interpersonal relationship with this new patient? What are some specific examples from the conversation that make you feel that way?

    _____
    _____
    _____
    _____

3. Do you think the sex of the patient and the sex of the provider might impact the information communicated? If so, why? If not, why not? Would your view change if the provider were a female and, as in this case, the patient a male?

    _____
    _____
    _____
    _____

4. What associated condition(s) for diabetics was/were not discussed during this inter-action that you think should have been covered? Why do you think it/they was/were not discussed?

    _____
    _____
    _____
    _____

Interactive Activity

- Rewrite (individually or in a group) the interaction between the provider and the patient.
- Try to discover a scenario that provides more information-sharing and relationship-building.
- Compare your rewrite to the Alternate Interaction that follows.

Interaction Rewrite

ALTERNATE INTERACTION
Insert your name and/or profession in the appropriate blanks below.

Mr. Santuli is seated in a chair in the examination room, dressed in his street clothes. The provider knocks on the door, enters the room, shakes the patient's hand, and pulls up a chair next to his.

Provider:	"Hi, Mr. Santuli. I'm _____, a _____."
Mr. Santuli:	"Hi, just call me Pietro."
Provider:	"Pietro, that's a great name. Is it Italian?"
Mr. Santuli:	"Yes, my family's from Naples."
Provider:	"My maiden name is Romeo; my grandparents came over from Milan."
Mr. Santuli:	"That's good; I was a little worried about having a new provider, but if you're Italian, that helps."
Provider:	"Well, I'm glad that helps, but I don't want you to be worried. Can we talk about what's bothering you?"
Mr. Santuli:	"I'm okay; they changed my insurance when I changed jobs, and they said I had to go to you."
Provider:	"I'm so sorry. How long were you with your previous provider?"
Mr. Santuli:	"I saw him for at least 15 years. Dr. Lunaci was Italian also."
Provider:	"I know Dr. Lunaci; what a nice man."
Mr. Santuli:	"Yeah, I was really upset that I had to stop seeing him. But you seem nice and the people at the front desk were nice."
Provider:	"Well, we try. So tell me, Pietro, how are you doing?"
Mr. Santuli:	"I'm doing okay; I wouldn't have come in except I need a new prescription, and my wife told me to."
Provider:	"Well, we can get you a new prescription, but why did your wife tell you to come see us?"
Mr. Santuli:	"I'm a little embarrassed to talk about it."
Provider:	"I understand. But I talk to patients all the time about their problems; do you want to try and talk to me about it?"
Mr. Santuli:	"I'm here, so I really don't want to come back, so here's the thing. Sometimes I can't get it up, and my wife thinks it's because of the sugar, and I think it's just that I'm getting old."

Provider: "Well, you might be right, but your wife could be right too. So we'll check your sugar, and if that's all under control, we'll get a urologist to see you and make sure that there isn't a prostate problem or some other cause for it. If not, then we can get you some medicine to help you get an erection. How's that sound?"

Mr. Santuli: "It sounds okay; so you're not going to examine me?"

Provider: "I'm going to examine you, but I'm going to let the urologist examine your prostrate and genitals."

Mr. Santuli: "Thanks."

Provider: "It's no problem; I completely understand. We'll get you the prescription refill and the consult with the urologist. Now, tell me about your diabetes and your high blood pressure."

Follow-up Discussion

1. How did the provider in the second scenario change the dynamic of the interaction? What specific verbal and nonverbal behaviors contributed to this change in the communication?

_____

_____

_____

_____

2. How did intercultural communication affect the exchange of information between the provider and patient?

_____

_____

_____

3. Do you agree with the provider's approach to minimizing the patient's discomfort with the situation? If so, why? If not, why not?

_____

_____

_____

4. How does the patient's condition impact his communication? How can providers help lessen patients' concerns in similar situations?

_____
_____
_____

5. In what ways can you envision current Health Maintenance Organization (HMO) or office management practices conflicting with the communication strategies used by the provider in the alternate scenario?

_____
_____
_____
_____

6. How did the provider in the alternate scenario work to build a relationship with the patient prior to discussing the patient's problem or concerns? Be specific.

_____
_____
_____
_____

7. How did the provider use the patient's feedback to help direct how she/he overcame his concerns and discomfort, and still get the information needed?

_____
_____
_____
_____

Key Points

1. Health communication differs from most other forms of interpersonal communication because of the unilateral emotional aspect of it. The patient is often upset, anxious, or fearful about his/her condition. Sometimes, that concern is increased because of cultural, social, or sexual taboos. Recognizing the problems that discussions about sex and sexual function present for patients and their families is critical for providers who want to increase information-exchange.

2. All too often patients are uncomfortable communicating the real reason for their visit. Consequently, providers need to recognize the importance of assessing a patient's nonverbal cues to see if the behaviors complement the verbal statements, or if there

are inconsistencies. Differences between verbal and nonverbal behaviors (e.g., no eye contact when talking) should be used by the provider as a sign that more inquiry is needed.

3. Relationship-building requires a bit more time on the provider's part, but the potential benefits exceed the cost. By encouraging conversation, providers have an opportunity to establish a relationship with the patient prior to and during the examination. By spending a few extra minutes developing an interpersonal relationship, the provider can enhance data collection, build trust, and increase the likelihood that the patient will be comfortable enough to discuss all his/her concerns.

4. Self-disclosure is a typical part of interpersonal communication. For most interpersonal relationships, however, self-disclosure signals trust between the communicators. Furthermore, self-disclosure by one person in a dyadic (two-person) conversation generally is expected to be reciprocated by the other person. However, in health communication, most interpersonal relationships do not involve mutual sharing of personal information, and providers are discouraged from self-disclosing intimate information to patients. Therefore, providers need to use their interpersonal communication skills to provide feedback to patients that illustrate the provider's recognition of the patient's self-disclosure, assure their confidentiality, and when necessary express their empathy without reciprocating.

I'VE GOT A DEFIBRILLATOR

18

Before reading the interaction below, please consider the following topics:

Media communication
- Mass media
  - Newspapers
  - Television
  - Magazines
  - Internet
- Media shape many people's views of healthcare
- Media decide what topics to cover, and in what depth
- Some media information, especially some internet sites, are not credible sources
- Media blur the distinction between what's news and what's presented as entertainment
- Media are driven by advertising sales that can be perceived as part of the news

Active listening
- Process for using as many senses as possible to enhance understanding
- Includes using feedback to assure accuracy
  - Paraphrasing what you heard to minimize misunderstanding
  - Both verbal and nonverbal communication
    - Asking questions
    - Nodding or shaking the head

INITIAL INTERACTION
Role play and/or analyze the following example:

Mary Camry is a 72-year-old female, who is seated in an Emergency Department cubicle. Her husband is seated on the gurney. The provider enters the cubicle and addresses Mr. Camry.

Provider: "Am I in the right room, or is your name Mary?"

Mr. Camry: "That's funny! No, that's Mary."

Provider: "Okay, neither of you look very ill, so why are you here?"

Ms. Camry: "I saw on the *Today* show that there was a recall of implanted defibrillators, and I have one, so I called my doctor's office and they said to come here."

Provider: "Okay, but it's 8 A.M.; if you'd waited until nine, I'm sure they'd be open and able to help you."

Ms. Camry: "Well, that's not what his office said, and I'm scared this thing is going to shock me—or not shock me. I don't know what to do, but I want you to take it out."

Provider: "That was an answering service you talked to, and they tell everyone with a problem to come here. But you don't know if you have a problem, and we don't take out implanted defibrillators here."

Ms. Camry: "I don't know about any of that. I just did what they said; now I want this thing out."

Provider: "Okay, you're not listening to me. Let's start over. What kind of defibrillator do you have?"

Ms. Camry: "I don't know."

Provider: "Didn't they give you a card with the information on it when they put it in?"

Ms. Camry: "I don't remember."

Provider: "I'm sure they gave you a card, and I'm sure they told you to carry it with you, in case you ever had a problem."

Ms. Camry: "Well, I don't have it and I don't remember any of that."

Provider: "Have you felt any shocks?"

Ms. Camry: "Oh my God, no!"

Provider: "That's good. How about any beeps—have you heard it beep?"

Ms. Camry: "You're really scaring me. Will it beep before it shocks me? Or will it just kill me? I just want this thing out!"

Provider: "It's not going to kill you; it's there to help you. Who is your cardiologist?"

Ms. Camry: "Dr. Conwell."

Provider:	"Okay, so you can go and give Dr. Conwell's office a call when you leave here and they'll get you an appointment."
Ms. Camry:	"You're not going to check it out, or take it out?"
Provider:	"Ma'am, I have no way to check it out, and we don't take them out in the Emergency Department. You haven't had any shocks or had a beep, and you don't know the make or model number of the defibrillator, so there's nothing I can do. Dr. Conwell can take care of this in a few minutes in his office."
Ms. Camry:	"But on TV they said it needed to be checked right away, and that it could be dangerous."
Provider:	"Well, they meant to check with your cardiologist. You were fine before you heard the news, so you'll be just fine till you get into Dr. Conwell's office."
Ms. Camry:	"I better be, 'cause my husband is a lawyer and he'll sue you and this hospital if anything happens."
Provider:	"I'll get your paperwork ready for you to check out."

Discussion Questions

1. How would you evaluate this communication exchange?

   _____

   _____

   _____

   _____

2. How would you have handled this patient's complaint—the same as in the scenario or differently, and why?

   _____

   _____

   _____

   _____

3. How did the media's reporting impact this communication?

   _____

   _____

   _____

4. How did the provider's attitude about the need for an Emergency Department visit alter the patient's perceptions of the interaction?

_____

_____

_____

_____

5. Do you feel that the patient's threat of legal action was justified? If so, how did the provider's communication impact the patient's threat? If not, why not?

_____

_____

_____

_____

Interactive Activity

- Rewrite (individually or in a group) the interaction between the provider and the patient.
- Try to discover a scenario that provides an outcome that is more acceptable to all members of the conversation.
- Compare your rewrite to the Alternate Interaction the follows.

Interaction Rewrite

_____

_____

_____

_____

_____

_____

_____

_____

_____

_____

_____

_____

_____

_____

ALTERNATE INTERACTION

Insert your name and/or profession in the appropriate blanks below.

Provider:	"Hi, Ms. Camry. I'm _____, and I'm a _____. What can I help you with today?"
Ms. Camry:	"I saw on the *Today* show that there was a recall of implanted defibrillators, and I have one, so I called my doctor's office and they said to come here."
Provider:	"I see; that must have been scary."
Ms. Camry:	"My husband thinks I'm crazy, but it scared me to death. I don't want to have this thing shock me or explode inside me."
Provider:	"I don't think you're crazy. I understand your fear. But the recall isn't because the defibrillators are exploding, so you can stop worrying about that. And only certain models are being recalled—do you know which model you have?"
Ms. Camry:	"No, I don't know which one it is."
Provider:	"Usually they give you a card with all the information about your defibrillator—do you remember getting one of the cards?"
Ms. Camry:	"No, I don't remember that and I don't have any card."
Provider:	"Okay, no problem. Let me ask you a couple of questions and listen to your heart, then we'll get an electrocardiogram and call your cardiologist."
Ms. Camry:	"You're not going to take it out?"
Provider:	"No, we don't do that here, but we'll make sure that everything's working okay, then we'll call your cardiologist to find out what model you have and what he or she wants us to do next."
Ms. Camry:	"He, Dr. Conwell—I tried to call him, but the office said to come here."
Provider:	"No problem. Have you felt any shocks from your defibrillator?"
Ms. Camry:	"No. Is it going to shock me?"
Provider:	"Well, it's made to shock your heart if the heart is beating unusually, but I'm just trying to get some information to give to Dr. Conwell. Have you ever heard the defibrillator beep?"
Ms. Camry:	"Oh my God, no! That would really scare me."
Provider:	"Okay, good. It sounds like your defibrillator is working normally, and I'll listen to your heart and we'll check the electrocardiogram, but I think everything is just fine."
Ms. Camry:	"I'm so glad to hear that, but I really think I'd be better off with it taken out. It just makes me so nervous."

Provider: "You should definitely talk to Dr. Conwell about that, but you've had it for a while, haven't you?"

Ms. Camry: "Almost a year."

Provider: "Well, you've been doing just fine with it for all that time, and it's probably helped to keep your heart beating normally, so you might want to keep it. Remember we don't even know if you have a model that is being recalled."

Ms. Camry: "So you think it's safe?"

Provider: "Let me finish my examination, but based on what we know, it seems very safe and very important for your health. I think you and Dr. Conwell need to have a discussion about it—but if you were my mom, I'd recommend you keep it in, and if it needs to be changed out because it's recalled, then I'd want you to get it changed out."

Ms. Camry: "That makes sense, and it makes me feel better to know you'd have your mother leave it in."

Provider: "I would, but I'd have her check with her cardiologist to see if she needs to have it changed. Now let's finish up, and I'll call Dr. Conwell as soon as we get the electrocardiogram and I listen to your heart."

Follow-up Discussion

1. How did the provider in the second scenario change the dynamic of the interaction? What specific verbal and nonverbal behaviors contributed to this change in the communication?

   _____

   _____

   _____

   _____

2. How did the provider use empathy and feedback to help calm the patient? What specific messages helped?

   _____

   _____

   _____

3. Do you agree with the provider's approach to minimizing the patient's fear? If so, why? If not, why not?

_____

_____

_____

4. Do you think the media is helpful when reporting recalls like this, or is there a better way to communicate this information to appropriate patients and their families?

_____

_____

_____

5. Would you have spent the time to call the patient's cardiologist or would you have told the patient to do it? If so, why? If not, why not?

_____

_____

_____

6. How did the provider in the alternate scenario work to build a relationship with the patient? Be specific.

_____

_____

_____

_____

7. Why do you think the patient did not threaten legal action in the second scenario?

_____

_____

_____

Key Points

1. Patients too often respond impulsively to information from the media, and health-care providers are ultimately where patients go to seek clarification and further information. Recalls of medicines and medical products cause patients and their families stress and concern, and their responses sometimes can be inappropriate. Providers need to recognize the cause of the patient's concern, and take the time to respond appropriately and to educate.

2. While it may seem unnecessary to see a patient in the Emergency Department for a non-life-threatening issue, providers have no choice but to try and educate the patient, and to help him/her find the appropriate source for follow-up care and discussion. In addition, our litigious society makes it risky to not evaluate a patient's concern and try to find an answer. It takes very little time to make a phone call to the patient's provider for information, but not doing so can result in unhappy patients and potential legal hassles.

3. All too often patients seek care, not for a problem, but for support. Active listening allows a provider to recognize the real reason for a visit, and to address the cause as well as the stated concern. By identifying the patient's fear, and educating and empowering the patient, a provider has a much greater opportunity for effective communication and a successful outcome.

4. Providers and patients often have similar goals, such as improving symptoms and maintaining or restoring health. However, many times providers and patients have disparate goals. For example, a provider may have a goal of reducing patient wait times, or increasing the number of patients seen in a day. While most patients prefer shorter wait times, that generally is not one of their goals, and clearly the number of patients a provider sees per day is not one of the patients' goals. Effective health communication allows providers and patients to have the best opportunity to attain all their goals—those that are similar and those that are unique to each.

I Saw This Ad on Television

19

Before reading the interaction below, please consider the following topics:

Gender communication
- Patients communicate differently based on their gender
  - Masculine-gendered individuals (male or female) tend to be more independent and not as communicative
  - Feminine-gendered patients (male or female) generally prefer to talk and express their concerns
- Providers need to recognize, based on a patient's gendered behaviors, if she/he is fully sharing information or getting the information they need

Direct-to-consumer advertising
- Because these advertisements are often interspersed among news programs, patients often perceive them as more factual than advertising
- Can help increase patient awareness about various medications and devices
- May require more conversation, clarification or explanation, on the provider's part, to address patient questions or requests generated by advertising

Negotiation
- Requires knowing what the other person wants and desires
- Providers should seek to understand what patients want, using open-ended rather than closed-ended questions
- Depends on providers and patients avoiding confrontation

INITIAL INTERACTION
Role play and/or analyze the following example:

Gordon Richards is sitting in the examination room as the provider enters. The 70-year-old man stands up and shakes hands with the provider.

Provider:	"How are you, Mr. Richards?"
Mr. Richards:	"I'm okay, how are you?"
Provider:	"I'm doing well; thanks for asking. What can I do for you today?"
Mr. Richards:	"I'm doing okay, and I'm not peeing as much as I used to."
Provider:	"How many times are you getting up during the night to urinate?"
Mr. Richards:	"One or two."
Provider:	"That's better than it was. Any other problems?"
Mr. Richards:	"No, not really. But I saw an ad on TV for this medicine; they said it's better than the one I'm taking. So do you think I should change?"
Provider:	"No; I put you on the prescription I thought would work best for you, and you're clearly doing better, so why would we want to switch?"
Mr. Richards:	"Well, my wife and I were talking, and the ad. just made the new medicine sound like it would work faster. So we thought I should ask."
Provider:	"That's their job to make it sound better in a commercial. I don't think it would work any better or faster. Let me see if your prostate has shrunk any on this medicine."
	(The provider does a rectal examination.)
Provider:	"Your prostate does feel a bit smaller than last time, so that's great—the medicine is working just fine."
Mr. Richards:	"And you don't think the other medicine would work better?"
Provider:	"If I thought the other medicine was better, I promise I would have put you on it. Now keep up the good work, and I'll see you in two months."
Mr. Richards:	"Okay, thanks."
	(After the provider leaves, Mr. Richards takes out his cell phone and dials his wife.)
Mr. Richards:	"I'm all done."
Mrs. Richards:	"How'd it go?"
Mr. Richards:	"He says I'm doing good and my prostate is smaller."
Mrs. Richards:	"Did you ask him about that new medicine?"
Mr. Richards:	"Yeah, he said I didn't need it."

Mrs. Richards:	"Did you tell him that they said it is better than the one you're on, and that Bernie is taking it and he's doing a lot better than you are?"
Mr. Richards:	"I told him. He wasn't very happy with me and I don't think he liked that I asked about it."
Mrs. Richards:	"Well, maybe you should go see Bernie's doctor."
Mr. Richards:	"I hate to start over with a new doctor, but I would like to sleep through the night."
Mrs. Richards:	"Me, too."

Discussion Questions

1. How would you react if you were the provider and the patient was pushing for a medicine from an advertisement over what you prescribed? Why do you feel that way?

_____

_____

_____

2. If you were the patient, how would you feel about the provider's response to your request?

_____

_____

_____

_____

3. How does direct-to-consumer (DTC) advertising impact your feelings and responses to patient requests for treatments other than the one(s) that were prescribed?

_____

_____

_____

_____

4. How do autonomy and power affect this provider–patient interaction?

_____

_____

_____

_____

5. If the provider had overheard the phone conversation between Mr. and Mrs. Richards, how do you think the provider would have reacted?

_____

_____

_____

_____

6. What do you think is the difference between the message the patient was sending and the message the provider heard?

_____

_____

_____

_____

7. How does the difference between denotative versus connotative meaning impact the communication that occurs in this scenario?

_____

_____

_____

_____

Interactive Activity

- Rewrite (individually or in a group) the interaction between the provider and the patient.
- What's your primary goal in creating a new scenario: enhancing the provider's credibility, complying with the patient's request, or better assessing the patient's concerns?
- Compare your rewrite to the Alternate Interaction that follows.

Interaction Rewrite

_____

_____

_____

_____

_____

_____

_____

ALTERNATE INTERACTION

Insert your name and/or profession in the appropriate blanks below.

The provider enters the examination room and goes over and shakes the patient's hand.

Provider:	"Hello, Mr. Richards. How're you doing today?"
Mr. Richards:	"I'm doing pretty good."
Provider:	"Okay, but you sound like you're concerned about something?"
Mr. Richards:	"I'm still getting up once or twice a night to pee, and it wakes my wife up and she can't go back to sleep, so she's not very happy with me."
Provider:	"I understand. I'm sure it's hard on her and on you. Losing sleep is never easy. But once or twice a night is much better than two or three times a night, right?"
Mr. Richards:	"Yes, but we saw this ad. on TV for this new medicine, and my wife thinks I should ask you if it would work better than the one I'm on."
Provider:	"Well, we can certainly discuss it. Let me examine your prostate and see if it's gotten any smaller. Then we can discuss the two medicines."
Mr. Richards:	"Okay."
	(The provider does a rectal examination.)
Provider:	"Your prostate is smaller, so the medicine you are on is working. But the other medicine you mentioned is very similar, so if you want to switch, we can try it. I'm just thinking that since the medicine you are now on is working—you're getting up less often at night and your prostate is smaller—then maybe we should just give it a little longer. But it's your decision, and I think you'll get better faster if you are comfortable with the medicine you are taking."
Mr. Richards:	"It's really okay with me, but my wife is the one who was most concerned."
Provider:	"Do you want me to talk with her?"
Mr. Richards:	"That would be great. She doesn't really trust me around doctors—she doesn't think I ask enough questions."
Provider:	"Do you want to call her now, or do you want her to call me later?"
Mr. Richards:	"If you don't mind, it would be easier on me if you could just talk to her now."
Provider:	"No problem, let's talk. Do you have a speaker on your phone? Or I can dial her on the office phone."
Mr. Richards:	"That would be great."
Provider:	"Hi, Mrs. Richards. This is _____. I was just talking to your husband and he wanted me to add you into our discussion, so you're on speaker phone."

Mrs. Richards:	"Hi, Gordon."
Mr. Richards:	"Hi, Emily. I mentioned the new medicine we saw on TV."
Provider:	"Yes, and that is a very good medicine. But what we were discussing is the fact that Mr. Richards' current medicine is working really well. He's going to the bathroom less frequently and his prostate has actually gotten smaller on the medicine. So everything seems to be going very well. But I understand that both of you are concerned about waking up during the night, and you wonder if the new medicine might work better. Is that correct?"
Mrs. Richards:	"Well, we have a friend, Bernie, who is taking it and he hardly ever gets up during the night."
Provider:	"That's great, and it might work that well for Mr. Richards too, but we don't know whether Bernie's prostate was as big as your husband's, or how his body responds to certain medicines differently than Mr. Richards' might. However, the new medicine you saw on TV is very similar to the one Mr. Richards is taking, so I'll be happy to change to that if that's what you two would like. I just suggested that we might want to give the current therapy two more months to see if it can eliminate the getting up at night to urinate. But if you both would prefer to switch now, rather than wait—I'll be happy to write a new prescription."
Mrs. Richards:	"Well, what do you think, Gordon?"
Mr. Richards:	"I think it makes sense to wait, if you don't mind?"
Mrs. Richards:	"It's up to you; I just wanted you better. So it's okay with me."
Provider:	"Good; then let's plan to see Mr. Richards in a month, and if things continue to improve, we'll recheck in another month. But if they aren't improving, then we'll try the new medicine. Is that okay with you both?"
Mrs. Richards:	"I'm okay with that."
Mr. Richards:	"Me, too. Thanks."

Follow-up Discussion

1. What are some of the key differences between the two scenarios?

   _____

   _____

   _____

2. How does the provider's willingness to talk to Mrs. Richards impact the outcome?

   _____

   _____

   _____

3. How do the extra few minutes on the phone affect the relationship between the provider and patient?

_____

_____

_____

4. How does the provider's self-concept and sense of autonomy differ in the two scenarios, and how might it have impacted the two interactions?

_____

_____

_____

5. How much does the patient's interpersonal communication with his wife contribute to the uncertainty in this scenario?

_____

_____

_____

6. Did the outcome of the second versus the first scenario make it worth the provider's time and effort? If so, why? If not, why not?

_____

_____

_____

7. How would you have handled the conversation from the provider's perspective—similarly or differently, and why?

_____

_____

_____

Key Points

1. Communication is continuous and interdependent, so the communication between the patient and his wife becomes integral to the provider–patient communication. The patient needs to make sure that his wife's questions are answered, but without effective communication between the provider and the patient, the provider will not be aware of the additional issues.

2. Gender differences (sex is determined by anatomy, but gender is related to psychological and sociological factors) frequently impact the provider–patient interaction. Feminine-gendered individuals are often more conversational, ask more questions, and seek collaboration. Masculine-gendered individuals (whether they are male or female),

on the other hand, tend not to ask many questions, to be more independent, and not to actively participate in their treatment decisions.

3. Providers who are willing to engage in a conversation about topics that are potential problems for patients may require a bit more time to accomplish their goals, but long-term can save time and the potential loss of patients. With the time constraints of modern medicine, there are a lot of compromises, but as this scenario illustrates, a few extra minutes can be the determining factor in keeping or losing a patient.

4. Compromise, rather than rejection or acquiescence, is often a very important communication strategy for provider–communicators. In this scenario, the provider could have done one of three things: refuse to change the prescription and risk losing the patient to a more accommodating provider; acquiesce and change to the new medicine, but risk an unhappy patient if the new medicine does not work as well as the original medicine; or offer to change, but suggest giving the new medicine a bit longer trial. With compromise, the patient and his wife in this case feel that they have a role in the decision-making, that their judgment is being given consideration, and that they understand the provider's rationale behind her/his treatment choice. Negotiation can be a very powerful tool in provider–patient interactions, but it requires providers to move away from an authoritarian, autonomous communication style, and embrace a more collaborative and participatory style.

EDUCATION
OR PROMOTION?
20

Before reading the interaction below, please consider the following topics:

Organizational communication
- Occurs within an organization, like a hospital or clinic
  - Includes the organization's mission, values, beliefs and policies, and how they are communicated to new and established employees
  - Impacts providers' communication with patients
- Occurs between organizations, like insurance companies and hospitals

Ethics
- Relies on providers conducting themselves with honor and integrity
- Depends on perceptions of others
- Ethical situations frequently result because of communication problems
  - More than one possible answer
  - No simple solution to the dilemma

INITIAL INTERACTION

Role play and/or analyze the following example:

Jane Allensworth is a sales representative for a pharmaceutical company. She's brought to the provider's office by a receptionist. The provider is seated behind the desk.

Provider:	"Hi, Jane. How are you doing?"
Ms. Allensworth:	"Hi, I'm fine, but how are you doing? From the look of that waiting room, your business is booming." (Laughter.)
Provider:	"We're keeping our heads above water. What can I do for you today?"
Ms. Allensworth:	"First, I brought you some samples; I'll put them in the closet. And I brought pizza and salad for the staff, so I hope you'll take a few minutes to grab a slice."
Provider:	"Thanks for the samples—we really do give them out to patients who don't have insurance. I think I'd better pass on the pizza, but I know the staff appreciates it when you bring lunch."
Ms. Allensworth:	"We're happy to do it; and I'll just need your signature for the samples."
Provider:	"No problem. Anything else I can do for you today?"
Ms. Allensworth:	"Are you still using our statin for your high cholesterol patients?"
Provider:	"Yep, I am. We've had pretty good luck with it, although I did have a couple of people recently with some myalgias, so we moved them over to your competitor."
Ms. Allensworth:	"How's that working out for you?"
Provider:	"So far, so good. Everybody seems happy with the change."
Ms. Allensworth:	"Did you try reducing the dose of our drug before switching them over? This graph shows how patients on a reduced dosage had fewer complaints."
Provider:	"I'll give it a try."
Ms. Allensworth:	"Okay, thanks. Now, how about I bring you a slice of pizza or some salad?"
Provider:	"Maybe I will do one slice and a small salad."

Discussion Questions

1. How did the sales representative use verbal communication to try and influence the provider?

   _____

   _____

   _____

   _____

2. What nonverbal behaviors did the sales representative use to try and impact the prescriber's perceptions of her product(s)?

   _____

   _____

   _____

   _____

3. From a health communication perspective, what is your perception of free lunches, samples, etc. on prescribing choices?

   _____

   _____

   _____

   _____

4. Do you think the provider has any ethical issues related to this conversation and his/her prescribing? If so, why? If not, why not?

   _____

   _____

   _____

   _____

5. How do you think patients, if they overheard this conversation, would perceive the message?

   _____

   _____

   _____

   _____

6. What do you think is the connotative meaning to the sales representative's message to the provider? What specific examples can you cite?

_____

_____

_____

_____

7. How would you assess this conversation between the provider and sales representative in terms of educational versus promotional goals and messages?

_____

_____

_____

_____

Interactive Activity

- Rewrite (individually or in a group) the interaction between the provider and the sales representative.
- Attempt to increase the educational aspect and minimize the promotional aspect of the conversation.
- Compare your rewrite to the Alternate Interaction that follows.

Interaction Rewrite

_____

_____

_____

_____

_____

_____

_____

_____

_____

_____

_____

_____

_____

_____

_____
_____
_____
_____
_____
_____
_____
_____
_____
_____
_____
_____
_____
_____
_____
_____
_____
_____

ALTERNATE INTERACTION

Provider:	"Hi, Jane. How are you doing?"
Ms. Allensworth:	"Hi, I'm okay; but the staff said you all don't want pizza?"
Provider:	"We've decided to stop accepting free food from sales representatives."
Ms. Allensworth:	"But you all have to eat and the staff seem to enjoy it."
Provider:	"I understand. But the providers had a meeting, and we think it's better for us and our patients if we stop the free stuff."
Ms. Allensworth:	"So what about samples?"

Provider:	"That was a big discussion as well. We are going to continue to accept samples, but we've changed our policy for distributing them, and they will be tightly controlled and only provided to new starts and patients who have insurance issues."
Ms. Allensworth:	"Okay. I'm a bit surprised, but whatever you all want to do is fine with me. Can I tell you about a recent study?"
Provider:	"Sure, but I'd prefer you leave me a copy of the paper."
Ms. Allensworth:	"Okay, I'll be happy to. Can I also leave you a little backgrounder on how we compare to other statins?"
Provider:	"No, I don't think I need that; let's just stick with the journal article."

Follow-up Discussion

1. What are some of the key differences between the two scenarios?

   _____

   _____

   _____

2. How do the changes in office policies impact the conversation?

   _____

   _____

   _____

3. In what ways do you think the changes in office policies will make maintaining an interpersonal relationship between the provider and sales representative more difficult?

   _____

   _____

   _____

4. Do you think the new policies make it more likely that future conversations between providers and sales representatives in the office will be more educational versus promotional?

   _____

   _____

   _____

   _____

5. Did the second conversation have more or less opportunity for confusion between the denotative and connotative meanings of the two communicators' conversations?

_____

_____

_____

_____

Key Points

1. Ethical issues are a part of all communication. Senders must be certain that their messages are clear and do not have any unethical connotations. In addition, receivers of messages need to analyze the communication to recognize any potentially questionable requests or improper requests or behaviors. While it is very nice to receive free lunches, as the old cliché goes: "nothing in life is truly free." There is an implied expectation that free food will enhance the provider–representative and office staff–representative relationship, which could lead to subconscious or even conscious prescribing decisions being influenced. In addition, by impacting the office staff, representatives may find it easier to gain access to providers.

2. Relationships between providers and sales representatives are different from relationships between providers and patients. The latter have similar goals of information-sharing in order to enhance the patient's health. The former have somewhat divergent goals, with the sales representative wanting to increase prescribing and the provider wanting to get information necessary to make treatment decisions. These diverse goals can lead to problems, especially in terms of how each interactant views the interpersonal communication and relationship with the other. Trying to recognize and critically assess your communication goals and those of the other person are very important to an effective and ethical information-exchange.

3. Providers clearly need information about new medications and treatments. However, there is a major difference between educational, peer-reviewed, nonbiased, clinical studies and promotional materials created by advertising and health education companies to persuade readers to prescribe a certain product. For providers, trying to ascertain the real facts about a particular medication or medical device can be difficult. However, when data are obfuscated by marketing and sales professionals, and then the financial ties of the authors are unclear or misrepresented, treatment decisions and conversations may be inaccurate, unethical, or inappropriate.

HOW ABOUT CEREAL FOR MY CHOLESTEROL?

21

Before reading the interaction below, please consider the following topics:

Compromise
- Strives for collaboration rather than competition
  - Decisions should be made through participation and mutual information-sharing
- Important to remember the key is to solve the patient's problem

Empowerment
- Allows patients to feel more in control of their lives
- Provides a sense of power
- Depends on knowledge
- Requires information-sharing and collaboration between patients and providers

Empathic Listening
- Requires focused listening
- Attempts to understand the other person's perceptions
- Lets patients talk about their problems without interrupting
- Enhances relationship-building

INITIAL INTERACTION

Role play and/or analyze the following example:

Wayne Nation is a 54-year-old white male, dressed and sitting in an examination room, waiting for the provider. Mr. Nation is being seen in follow-up to his annual physical examination. The provider enters the room and sits down opposite Mr. Nation.

Provider:	"Mr. Nation, how are you today?"
Mr. Nation:	"I'm okay. How were the blood tests?"
Provider:	"You sound like you are in a hurry."
Mr. Nation:	"I'm not in a hurry; but you scared me last week when you did my physical. I really don't want to take medicine."
Provider:	"Okay, your lab results look pretty good. Your blood count was normal, and your electrolytes, kidney and liver function, and prostate tests are all normal. But your cholesterol is high, and you have too much bad cholesterol and not enough good cholesterol."
Mr. Nation:	"Well, that sounds bad."
Provider:	"It's not bad, but like we discussed last time, if your numbers weren't better than last year, you'll need to get on medications."
Mr. Nation:	"I've made it 54 years without taking any medicines every day, so I'm really not big on starting now."
Provider:	"Well, you've done pretty well, but you need to be on a baby aspirin every day, and since changing your diet and exercise didn't lower your numbers very much, you should be on a statin for your cholesterol."
Mr. Nation:	"What if I exercise and diet more?"
Provider:	"You told me you'd been exercising for the past six months and you'd lost 10 pounds on Weight Watchers, didn't you?"
Mr. Nation:	"Yes, but I saw a commercial that if I eat cereal, my cholesterol will go down. How about if I eat several bowls a day, and then we recheck it?"
Provider:	"Those commercials are only trying to sell you cereal; they aren't going to lower your cholesterol like a statin, and you'll be putting on weight at the same time—which isn't good for your heart, blood pressure, back, knees, etc. No, I think you need to stop paying attention to TV and listen to me. You need to be on a low dose statin and a baby aspirin every day."
Mr. Nation:	"I hear what you're saying, but it's my body and I'm going to try the cereal first."

Discussion Questions

1. What issues did you have with this conversation and its outcome?

_____

_____

_____

_____

2. How could the provider have approached the patient differently and achieved a more mutually acceptable outcome? Be specific.

_____

_____

_____

_____

3. How would you handle a patient who does not want to follow your advice or treatment recommendation?

_____

_____

_____

_____

4. For a patient who clearly wants to avoid taking medications, can you come up with a different strategy?

_____

_____

_____

_____

5. How would you use health communication and education to try and overcome the patient's objections and achieve a different outcome?

_____

_____

_____

_____

Interactive Activity

- Rewrite (individually or in a group) the interaction between the provider and the patient.
- Attempt to educate and empower the patient.
- Compare your rewrite to the Alternate Interaction that follows.

Interaction Rewrite

ALTERNATE INTERACTION

Provider: "Hi, Mr. Nation; it's great to see you again."

Mr. Nation: "Hi. I wish I could say I was happy to see you, but I'm really worried about the blood test results."

Provider: "I'm sorry you are worried. Your results were pretty good, but we've got to talk about the cholesterol."

Mr. Nation: "I really don't want to take medicine. Once my father started taking medicine, his health just went downhill and he was dead in a year or two."

Provider: "I'm so sorry about your father, but I can tell you from my experiences that almost all of my patients who take a cholesterol-lowering medicine do very well. And as we discussed last time, you should be on a baby aspirin every day, especially with your family history."

Mr. Nation: "What if I eat more cereal? I saw some commercials that show it can lower my cholesterol."

Provider: "Well, I've seen those commercials and they say they can lower your cholesterol four or five percent, but for you—with cholesterol of 262—that's only about 10 points, and we need to get yours down more than 60 points. And even more importantly, we need to try and get your HDL, the good cholesterol, higher and your LDL, the bad cholesterol, lower. But your triglycerides are normal, so that's good."

Mr. Nation: "Wow, 60 points! And you don't think dieting and exercise, with some cereal too, will get it down enough?"

Provider: "I really don't. You told me last week that you'd been exercising and dieting, and we know you've lost 10 pounds since last year, but your cholesterol only went down 15 points from last year and it's still high. So I don't think it's realistic to believe you're going to be able to significantly lower your cholesterol by diet and exercise alone."

Mr. Nation: "Can I try it? I will really work on a diet; I'll even get a personal trainer at the gym—I just don't want to take medicine."

Provider: "Did you read the pamphlet I gave you last week about cholesterol and how it can build up in your blood vessels if it's not controlled?"

Mr. Nation: "I did, and I understand that it's probably why my father died at 63, but he smoked and ate like a horse."

Provider: "You know, it's your decision; I just want to make sure you understand the realities of having high cholesterol. No one can tell you how long it's safe to put off taking medicines that will lower your cholesterol, but we can show you statistics regarding the risk of high cholesterol over time. What if we compromise? You take a baby aspirin—that's not a prescription medicine and it's something you really do need to be taking every day—and then try your cereal, diet, and exercise for three months. Then we'll recheck your numbers in three months, and you agree that if they are still high, that you'll take a statin. Will that work for you?"

Mr. Nation: "I can do that. I'm not crazy about taking the aspirin, but it's not a prescription, and I will really work on my diet and exercise and do the cereal every day and see if I can't get it down. I don't want to have a heart attack, but I don't want to be on a bunch of medicines if I can avoid them."

Follow-up Discussion

1. What are some of the key differences between the two scenarios?

   _____

   _____

   _____

2. How does the provider's willingness to listen to the patient's concerns impact the outcome?

   _____

   _____

   _____

   _____

3. Do you agree with the provider's compromise? If so, why? If not, why not?

   _____

   _____

   _____

4. What do you think would have happened if the provider had refused to compromise and forced the patient to take a prescription for a statin?

   _____

   _____

   _____

   _____

5. How do the patient's psychological concerns about taking medicines change the focus of the conversation?

_____

_____

_____

_____

6. How did the provider empower the patient to make an informed decision? Be specific.

_____

_____

_____

_____

Key Points

1. Providers have an obligation to provide the most accurate information they can to patients. In addition, providers need to be assured that patients understand the information, and to answer any questions. However, adults who are intellectually capable of analyzing and assessing the information they receive often want the power to make informed decisions.

2. Not all outcomes can result in patients agreeing fully with their providers, or complying with the providers' recommendations or treatment decisions. Sometimes outcomes need to be negotiated in a way that provides the patient with the best opportunity for a successful outcome.

3. The media have an ever-increasing role in health communication, and part of the empowerment efforts of providers is to help patients interpret the information provided on television, online, and via print media. Patients often lose sight of the fact that the goal of marketing is to sell products—not to educate. Providers have to serve as an education resource for patients and present diverse views so patients can be empowered to make informed treatment decisions. For many providers, the time it takes to educate patients and present the information is very time-consuming. However, the power of marketing requires additional efforts to educate and overcome the one-sided view presented in the media.

ARE VACCINES SAFE?

22

Before reading the interaction below, please consider the following topics:

Communicating with parents
- Parents need and want clear information about their child's illness, injury, or health status
- Parents must make healthcare decisions for their children
  - That can cause anxiety and stress
- Providing parents with written materials about the child's condition, diagnosis, or treatment is often extremely helpful
- Assess the health literacy level of parents in order to communicate effectively in person or in written documents
- Don't forget to communicate with the pediatric patient
  - Relationship-building, even with young children, can help reduce fear and enhance trust

Written communication
- Can be used to help answer questions that arise after an interaction
- Must be written at the health literacy level of the patient or family member
- Whenever possible, should be supplied prior to meeting with the provider to help address any concerns or stimulate any remaining questions
- Useful in countering inaccurate information on the Internet or from friends and/or relatives
- Should be kept concise and clear
  - Use bullets for key points
  - Avoid medical or technical jargon

INITIAL INTERACTION

Role play and/or analyze the following example:

Karen Herbee is the mother of a one-year-old child, Caitlin, who is at the pediatrician's office for her check-up and her vaccinations. The provider has just finished Caitlin's examination.

Provider:	"As I'm sure you gathered, everything looks great today, so we'll be giving her the flu vaccine."
Ms. Herbee:	"I'm a little worried about that. Doesn't it have mercury in it?"
Provider:	"It's such a small amount after they do the filtering, that it's only a trace."
Ms. Herbee:	"But I've been reading in the paper that a lot of people think vaccines cause autism."
Provider:	"There's no research that shows that, and they've done several studies."
Ms. Herbee:	"I heard there was a spray type."
Provider:	"There is, but it's only for children 5 years and older."
Ms. Herbee:	"I really don't think I'll have her get it then."
Provider:	"That's your choice, but I'd recommend she have it. The flu is dangerous in small children, and like I said, there's no scientific evidence that thimerosal causes any problems."
Ms. Herbee:	"Well, I've talked to parents of autistic children and they say they started to notice a change after the vaccinations."
Provider:	"I understand, but autism usually isn't diagnosed until a child is 2 or 3—and that's after the vaccinations—but that doesn't mean the vaccinations caused it. As I said, there are lots of studies that show no causal link. But if you don't want the flu vaccine, that's your choice, but I do want to advise you that you are making that decision against medical advice."
Ms. Herbee:	"Well, that's not the only decision I'm making today. We'll just hold off on all her shots, and I'll find another pediatrician."
Provider:	"That's your choice, but you'll need to sign a records release form."

Discussion Questions

1. How would you evaluate the communication in this scenario?

   _____

   _____

   _____

   _____

2. What is your view of the provider's education of the mother regarding her daughter's vaccination?

   _____

   _____

   _____

   _____

3. What do you think would have helped assure a more positive outcome for this interaction, from both the provider's and mother's perspectives?

   _____

   _____

   _____

   _____

4. What would you have done differently to enhance the health communication exchange in this scenario? Be specific.

   _____

   _____

   _____

   _____

5. How do you view provider–parent interactions differently from provider–patient communication?

   _____

   _____

   _____

   _____

6. Do you agree that the need for influenza immunization is more important than the mother's concerns and/or the risk of problems with a trace of thimerosal in the vaccine?

_____

_____

_____

_____

7. How do you think the media and innuendo have impacted parents' attitudes and concerns about vaccines and the risk of autism? How can you, as a provider, prepare for these types of discussions?

_____

_____

_____

_____

Interactive Activity

- Rewrite (individually or in a group) the interaction between the provider and the patient or parent of the patient.
- Rewrite the conversation, and try to improve the communication effectiveness and interpersonal relationship between the provider and the child's mother.
- Compare your rewrite to the Alternate Interaction that follows.

Interaction Rewrite

_____

_____

_____

_____

_____

_____

_____

_____

_____

_____

_____

_____

ALTERNATE INTERACTION

Provider: "Okay, Caitlin, that's all the poking and pushing. She's doing just great and her examination is completely normal today, so I think we're ready to give her those vaccinations. Did you get a chance to read over the Centers for Disease Control and Prevention (CDC) information sheets we gave you at the last visit about today's flu vaccine?"

Ms. Herbee: "I did, but I'm still nervous about the thimerosal in the flu shot."

Provider: "That's a perfectly understandable feeling. Can you tell me about your concerns?"

Ms. Herbee: "Well, I know what the handout said and I understand that they did studies, but I know people and I've heard stuff on the radio and read things in magazines that make it sound like they may be trying to cover something up, or they just don't know."

Provider: "Those are very valid concerns and it's worrisome to all of us how many children are diagnosed with autism. However, we all have to try and look at the science and compare it to rumors and conjecture. They have done a lot of research on this and no one has been able to find a direct link."

Ms. Herbee: "What about that study in England? Didn't they say there was a link?"

Provider: "They suggested that there might be a need for more studies, because they found some mercury in some of their patients, but even they said they couldn't be sure it was because of thimerosal. And while your concerns make perfect sense, you have to weigh the risk versus Caitlin getting the flu, and becoming dehydrated and requiring hospitalization, etc."

Ms. Herbee: "The flu just seems like such a small thing compared to autism."

Provider: "There is no question that flu in healthy, young adults is mostly an inconvenience, but in small children like Caitlin, and in the elderly who Caitlin might give it to if she gets it—the flu can be devastating."

Ms. Herbee: "I hate that we have to make a decision that could end up making her sick, or causing her to be autistic for the rest of her life."

Provider: "I assure you, that if I—or any other pediatric provider—thought there was any chance that this would cause Caitlin or any child to be autistic, we'd never recommend it. But all the data show that the vaccine and thimerosal do not cause autism. What does your husband think of all this?"

Ms. Herbee: "He's a man! He thinks I'm being silly. He says we took the vaccines when we were children and they didn't cause us any problems, so I shouldn't be so worried."

Provider: "Well, I don't agree that you shouldn't think about this carefully, and it's normal to be concerned. But I do agree that vaccines have been used for decades with great success and saved countless lives and suffering."

Ms. Herbee: "I saw on the form you gave me to read that there's a thimerosal-free flu vaccine, and it said to talk to you about it?"

Provider: "Yes, there is; however, it's not widely stocked. We don't have any of it, and I've tried to find it for some other parents and I've had no luck. But I'll tell you what I told them—you may want to call around to the hospitals and other doctors' offices to see if anyone has any. If you find it, we'll be happy to administer it."

Ms. Herbee: "Thanks, but I guess if you and my husband and the CDC think it's safe, then I'll stop worrying about it."

Provider: "I think you're making the right decision, but I want to make sure you are comfortable with it. Do you want to come back later, and talk more with your husband, or try to locate the thimerosal-free vaccine?"

Ms. Herbee: "No, I'm convinced. I just wanted to talk with you about it, and I am so grateful that you took the time to talk with me and didn't make me feel like I was an idiot for worrying."

Provider: "You're not an idiot! You're Caitlin's mom and you're trying to do what you think is best for her health. That's exactly what we want all parents to do. I respect your concern and I applaud your researching it and discussing it. Now any questions, or shall we give Caitlin her shots and get you all on your way?"

Ms. Herbee: "Let's get her vaccinated and then I'll get her something to eat."

Follow-up Discussion

1. What are some of the key communication differences between the two scenarios? Be specific.

    _____

    _____

    _____

    _____

2. Have you ever provided patients with handouts or educational information *in advance* of a visit, so they can prepare questions and do additional research? If so, why? If not, why not?

    _____

    _____

    _____

    _____

3. How would you assess the communication effectiveness of the second versus the first interaction?

_____

_____

_____

4. How much more time, if any, do you think the second scenario would have taken compared to the first? If more, do you think it was worth it?

_____

_____

_____

5. How do you think the provider's questions about Caitlin's dad and his feelings about the vaccine, and the provider's suggestion that her mom try to find thimerosal-free vaccine impacted the outcome of the alternate scenario?

_____

_____

_____

_____

_____

Key Points

1. Communicating with parents, especially of small children, can require more time and empathy. Parents often want to spend more time than they do as patients themselves, discussing their child's condition and treatment plans. In addition, with the explosion of information on the Internet, parents have frequently done research at a wide variety of websites—some credible and some not—but seek further information from the healthcare provider. They generally want reassurance that as parents they are doing everything they can to protect their child's health. Therefore, providers need to recognize this fairly unique communication setting. The pediatric patient cannot verbalize or can minimally verbalize his/her problems and/or symptoms or questions, and the parent serves the role of advocate and decision-maker. Providers must recognize how difficult this role is for some parents, and how much stress seemingly innocent decisions like vaccinations and circumcisions can cause. Parents are deciding whether to let their children have procedures or immunizations in the hope that they will improve health or decrease complications later in life. At the same time, parents often recognize that a child, who is healthy, may suffer some unintended consequences from the parents' decision-making. Education, empowerment, and empathy are important communication skills to utilize in

helping parents recognize the provider's desire to help the parent reach the best outcome for the pediatric patient.

2. The media have become a major factor in provider–patient and provider–parent interactions. With topics like vaccines and their relationship or nonrelationship to the development of autism, radio talk-show hosts, internet blogs, newspaper articles, television news shows, etc. compete with published clinical studies and reports from governmental agencies like the National Institutes of Health (NIH) and the CDC. Providers need to be well informed, not only about the most recent studies on various topics affecting their patients, but also about what is being said in the lay media. By providing patients and parents with handouts from credible organizations that can be reviewed, especially in advance if possible, the provider encourages the patient or parent to research, assimilate, and discuss his/her concerns, assessments, or questions. Providers need to try and make certain that patients, and especially parents, have scientific information to assess versus the often nonscientific media information they are receiving. The more informed the patient or parent is, the better chance a provider has at sharing ideas, empowering, and continuing to build a relationship.

THE ROLE OF THIRD PARTIES IN HEALTH COMMUNICATION

IV

HOW SAFE
ARE GENERICS?
23

Before reading the interaction below, please consider the following topics:

Organizational communication
- Organizations communicate with their employees, vendors, and customers
    - In healthcare, countless organizations must communicate with a variety of audiences
        - For example, the Food and Drug Administration (FDA) must communicate with
            - Pharmaceutical companies
            - Physicians
            - Physician Assistants (PAs) and Advance Practice Registered Nurses (APRNs)
            - Hospitals
            - Pharmacists
- For economic reasons, health insurance companies communicate on a regular basis with
    - Providers
    - Pharmacists
    - Patients
    - Hospitals
- It's important to remember that each organization has its own goals, values, and beliefs; sometimes these goals are divergent and can cause conflicts in communication and decision-making

Patient empowerment

- Depends on information-sharing
- For patients or parents to be in control, they need to understand the situation and the possible choices
- The Internet may be a good source for information, but it depends on the site
  - Can assist patients with known credible sources of information beyond themselves
    - Through written handouts
    - Via trusted online sources
- The patient's or family's health literacy must be assessed and taken into account by the provider

INITIAL INTERACTION

Role play and/or analyze the following example:

Caroline Bettis is a 33-year-old stock broker, who is being treated for hypothyroidism following thyroid ablation with I_{131}. She has come to see the provider for a routine follow-up examination.

Provider:	"Hi, Ms. Bettis. How are you doing today?"
Ms. Bettis:	"I'm good. How were the tests?"
Provider:	"Your lab. tests look great, so we're going to get you started on thyroid replacement medicine."
Ms. Bettis:	"And I have to take that forever?"
Provider:	"Yes, we ablated your thyroid and now we've got to give you medicine to replace the hormone it produces."
Ms. Bettis:	"Well, that sounds scary."
Provider:	"No, we do it all the time. Your examination and your tests are good, so here's a prescription for thyroid hormones."
Ms. Bettis:	"What's Levothyroxine?"

Provider:	"That's the generic name of the thyroid medicine."
Ms. Bettis:	"Isn't there a brand-name drug you can give me?"
Provider:	"I can, but they'll just change it to a generic. Insurance companies won't pay for brand-name drugs for thyroid replacement, so it's a generic."
Ms. Bettis:	"Do they work? I thought I read something about them not working as well as the brand-name one?"
Provider:	"The FDA says they work and they're safe. Plus, it's not like you have a lot of choices, unless you want to pay for it out of your own pocket."
Ms. Bettis:	"It makes me nervous that I'm taking a generic."
Provider:	"I wouldn't worry; lots of medicines are generics these days. The insurance companies make sure we get the cheapest pills possible."

Discussion Questions

1. What issues did you have with this conversation?

    _____

    _____

    _____

    _____

2. How could the provider have approached the patient differently and made her feel more comfortable with the situation? Be specific.

    _____

    _____

    _____

    _____

3. How would you handle a patient who is nervous about taking a generic versus a brand-name medication?

    _____

    _____

    _____

    _____

4. Which provider language choices do you find troubling, and why?

_____

_____

_____

_____

5. How would you use health communication and education to try and overcome the patient's concerns?

_____

_____

_____

_____

Interactive Activity

- Rewrite (individually or in a group) the interaction between the provider and the patient.
- Use your interpersonal communication and relationship-building skills to help educate the patient and minimize her concerns.
- Compare your rewrite to the Alternate Interaction that follows.

Interaction Rewrite

_____

_____

_____

_____

_____

_____

_____

_____

_____

_____

_____

_____

_____

_____

_____

_____

_____

_____

_____

_____

_____

_____

_____

_____

_____

_____

_____

_____

_____

_____

_____

ALTERNATE INTERACTION

Provider:	"Hi, Ms. Bettis. How are you feeling today?"
Ms. Bettis:	"Hi. I'm okay, but how are my tests?"
Provider:	"They show just what we expect. Since we treated your thyroid, it's not producing thyroid hormone in the high amounts like it was when you first came in. So the radioactive iodine that you took did its job."
Ms. Bettis:	"So now what happens?"

Provider: "Well, we need to get you started on some thyroid replacement medicine. As we talked about before, your body needs thyroid hormones, but not in large doses like you were getting. So we'll start you out on a low dose of replacement medicine, and recheck your lab. tests and adjust the dose up or down as needed."

Ms. Bettis: "Will the medicine make me sick, or make my heart race like it did before?"

Provider: "No, it shouldn't. We're going to start with a low dose and we'll gradually increase it as needed. But keep in mind, this is a process, and it may take several months until we find just the right dose to regulate your thyroid hormone level in your blood."

Ms. Bettis: "So can I get a mail order prescription?"

Provider: "No, we don't want to do that yet, because they only do a three-month supply, and until we know the dose that we'll keep you at, we'll likely be changing the prescription monthly. But it's a generic, so it's not very expensive."

Ms. Bettis: "I don't think I've ever taken a generic. I don't even buy generic canned vegetables—do they work? And how safe are generics?"

Provider: "Well, I don't know about generic canned vegetables, but I can tell you that the FDA has to approve a generic, just like it does a brand-name medicine. So yes, they work; I have lots of patients on generics—and the FDA says they are safe. I can order a brand-name thyroid medicine instead of the generic, but I'm guessing your insurance company will make the pharmacist use the generic."

Ms. Bettis: "Do you have any information on generics that I could read?"

Provider: "I'm sorry, I don't, but you can get on the Internet and go to the Generic Pharmaceutical Association, www.gphaonline.org, or www.fda.gov, and read all about generics there. And the pharmacist will likely have some information too."

Ms. Bettis: "Okay, that's good; I just like to know as much as I can about the medicines I'm putting into my body."

Provider: "That makes sense to me. And remember, you can ask the pharmacist for the brand-name medicine, but you'll have to pay the difference."

Follow-up Discussion

1. What are some of the key differences between the two scenarios?

   _____

   _____

   _____

2. How does the provider's willingness to discuss generic medicine help build a relationship between the patient and provider?

_____

_____

_____

_____

_____

3. What role does the insurance company play in the interaction between the patient and the provider?

_____

_____

_____

_____

4. Since there are differing views on consistency of generic versus brand-name thyroid replacement drugs, how do you think the provider should present the information to the patient?

_____

_____

_____

_____

_____

5. How do the differing views on generic thyroid medicines among some medical associations, generic manufacturers, and the FDA impact the patient's education by the provider and their decision-making?

_____

_____

_____

_____

6. Do you agree with the way the provider communicated information about the topic to the patient? If so, why? If not, why not?

_____

_____

_____

_____

Key Points

1. Patients need to know as much as possible about their diseases and potential treatment options. Sometimes that requires educating them about controversies among providers, associations, and/or government agencies. Patients rely on their providers to be well informed on these topics. However, in order to empower patients and build a relationship, providers need to determine how much information about controversial issues the patients and their families need, and not only provide it, but identify sources where further material can be accessed, like credible websites.

2. Today third parties are frequently involved in treatment decisions. The role of case managers, insurers, etc. has added an additional layer of communication to the provider–patient decision-making process. Therefore, it frequently reduces the provider's time to discuss with patients in advance how third parties may impact decisions about various treatment modalities.

3. Patients frequently bring their everyday notions of brand-name versus generic products to their discussions of generic medications. Therefore, providers have to help educate patients about current information regarding how generic medicines are similar to and/or different from brand-name medications. The more providers can educate themselves about FDA standards and current thinking among thought-leaders and professional associations, about the differences between generic and brand-name treatments for specific diseases, the easier it will be to have discussions with patients.

I Can't Work

24

Before reading the interaction below, please consider the following topics:

Third party communication
- Health communication frequently requires communication with parties other than the patient
  - Family members
  - Other providers
  - Insurers
  - Employers (for worker's compensation cases)
- Third parties frequently have different needs and goals from the patient and the provider
- Health Insurance Portability and Accountability Act (HIPAA) requirements restrict some conversations without the patient's approval

Trust
- Necessary for developing effective interpersonal relationships
- Key for negotiations between providers and patients or their families
- Important to realize that authority figures, like healthcare providers, can be perceived as threatening or trying to control the situation or interaction
- Required because providers need to be viewed as credible and trustworthy if they are to empower patients and collaborate in decision-making

INITIAL INTERACTION

Role play and/or analyze the following example.
Insert your name and/or profession in the appropriate blanks below.

Carl Low is a 27-year-old construction worker, who is leaning against the counter in the examination room as the provider enters the door.

Provider: "Mr. Low, good morning. I'm _____, a _____; what's going on today?"

Mr. Low: "Hi. I hurt my shoulder at work and it's really killing me."

Provider: "How'd you hurt it?"

Mr. Low: "I was carrying some lumber on my shoulder and walking up a ramp, and I guess I just slipped off the side, 'cause I tumbled to the ground and the wood fell on my shoulder."

Provider: "So when did this happen?"

Mr. Low: "It happened last night, and I went to the ER and they did an X-ray and said it wasn't broken and to come here."

Provider: "Okay, and it still hurts today?"

Mr. Low: "Yeah, it's killing me."

Provider: "Okay, so where does it hurt?"

Mr. Low: "Right here, on top of the shoulder, and it really hurts when I try to raise it up."

Provider: "Okay, so show me how high you can lift your arm."

Mr. Low: "That's it."

Provider: "Now, relax and let me try to raise it a bit higher."

Mr. Low: "Ow! It won't go any higher!"

Provider: "All right, so we'll order an MRI of your shoulder."

Mr. Low: "Will they do that today?"

Provider: "No, they have to get the Worker's Compensation insurance to approve it, and that can take a few days."

Mr. Low: "That sucks; so what am I supposed to do in the meantime?"

Provider: "I have no control over the insurance company, but we'll get you light duty and some pain medicine."

Mr. Low: "I can't work! I can't even raise my arm."

Provider: "Light duty means you won't use your arm; you'll be restricted to only working with your left arm."

Mr. Low: "You're kidding, right? Have you ever done construction? There's no light duty."

Provider: "Then they have to send you home. But my job is to tell them what you can do, and it's up to them to find a job that meets those requirements or send you home."

Discussion Questions

1. How would you evaluate the communication in this scenario?

   _____

   _____

   _____

   _____

2. What third parties are impacting this communication? How are they affecting it?

   _____

   _____

   _____

3. Do you think it should be the provider's role to educate the patient about the Worker's Compensation process? If so, why? If not, why not?

   _____

   _____

   _____

   _____

4. What do you think are the implications for treatment decisions, based on the various third parties' roles in this case?

   _____

   _____

   _____

   _____

5. As third parties become more involved in treatment decisions, how do you think a provider's interpersonal communication with patients will need to adapt?

   _____

   _____

   _____

   _____

6. How might your interpersonal relationship with a patient be reduced by third parties' roles in treatment decisions, timing, etc.?

   _____

   _____

   _____

   _____

7. What do you see as a potential setback to the patient's prognosis, based on this scenario and conversation.

_____

_____

_____

_____

Interactive Activity

- Rewrite (individually or in a group) the interaction between the provider and the patient.
- Rewrite the conversation, and try to improve the communication effectiveness and interpersonal relationship between the provider and the patient.
- Compare your rewrite to the Alternate Interaction that follows.

Interaction Rewrite

_____

_____

_____

_____

_____

_____

_____

_____

_____

_____

_____

_____

_____

_____

_____

_____

_____

_____

_____
_____
_____
_____
_____
_____
_____
_____
_____
_____
_____
_____
_____
_____
_____
_____
_____
_____
_____
_____

ALTERNATE INTERACTION

Insert your name and/or profession in the appropriate blanks below.

Provider: "Hello, Mr. Low. I'm _____, a _____. I see you're in pain—what happened?"

Mr. Low: "Hi. I was carrying a load of lumber up a ramp; it was on my shoulder, and I somehow fell off the ramp and the lumber landed on my shoulder?"

Provider: "Okay, then what happened?"

Mr. Low: "I went to the ER, and they X-rayed me and said nothing was broken, but it's really hurting me."

Provider: "Sorry, but did you hit your head when you fell?"

Mr. Low:	"No, just hurt my shoulder."
Provider:	"Okay, I have a few more questions, then I'll examine you and we'll talk about next steps. But first, have you ever had a Worker's Compensation injury before?"
Mr. Low:	"No, this is my first. Why?"
Provider:	"Well, it makes a difference in how things are done—I want you to know in advance, because most people think it's just like with your health insurance, but it's not. So here's what happens: you'll see me every week and my job is to help you get well, but I also have to tell your company what work you can and can't do. Also, I have to tell the Worker's Compensation insurance company how you're doing, what tests we need, and what treatments I want you to have. So unlike most health insurance companies, where we order the tests and they bill them, we can't get anything done without getting approvals first, and sometimes that takes a few days. I just want to make sure you understand the process, so you don't get frustrated, or think we're not working as fast as possible."
Mr. Low:	"Sounds like it's a real pain."
Provider:	"It's occasionally a bit slower than any of us would like. Now, let's finish your examination, and then we'll talk about what we need to do next."
Mr. Low:	"Would it help if I called them?"
Provider:	"Sometimes it helps because they may have questions about the accident, or it gets delayed for other reasons, so I would encourage you to talk with the case manager at your Worker's Compensation insurance company."

Follow-up Discussion

1. What are some of the key differences between the two scenarios?

   _____

   _____

   _____

   _____

2. How does the provider's discussion of the Worker's Compensation process impact the provider–patient interaction?

   _____

   _____

   _____

   _____

3. Do you think it was worth the provider's time to educate the patient about the process? If so, why? If not, why not?

_____

_____

_____

_____

4. Do you think the provider's discussion of the process was biased or unbiased toward the process and the third parties? Do you agree with this approach? If so, why? If not, why not?

_____

_____

_____

_____

5. How would you feel as a patient if you knew that there were multiple third parties involved in your treatment decisions?

_____

_____

_____

_____

Key Points

1. There are many instances in healthcare today where parties beyond the provider and patient are involved in, or impact the communication with and/or treatment of patients. From health departments to insurance companies, and to employers in Worker's Compensation, numerous outside influences affect the communication and decision-making of providers and patients. Therefore, it's important for providers to make patients aware of the process, to minimize any misunderstanding and frustration. Too often, when patients do not receive the diagnostic tests and/or treatments that the provider ordered, the patient blames the provider or his/her office staff for the delay or changes. Communicating the process in advance helps to improve understanding, but also empowers the patient to take a more active role in contacting the appropriate person as the third party, to help facilitate the process.

2. As we know, trust is critical to the development and maintenance of an interpersonal relationship. In this scenario, the patient has an injury that will likely take multiple visits over weeks or months to heal, so the provider and patient need to work together to assure a successful outcome. By taking a few minutes to educate and empower patients about the process and how it is impacted by third parties,

providers can build trust and enhance communication. Providers should assess the potential value of spending a few minutes discussing the role of third parties, when appropriate, versus having to deal with a frustrated, unhappy patient later.

3. Working with patients is a partnership. While it is true that most of the time the provider knows more about diagnosing and treating a patient's illness or injury, providers still need patients to get needed tests, follow treatment regimens, etc. In today's healthcare system, the role of third parties in patient care and treatment impacts not just the patient, but also the provider–patient communication. Therefore, providers need to educate patients about the process in order to improve the partnership, minimize frustration, and enhance compliance.

You'll Feel Better Recovering at Home
25

Before reading the interaction below, please consider the following topics:

Communication roles
- Providers must assume a number of communication roles
  - Information source
  - Information gatherer
  - Empathic listener
  - Medical expert
  - Team leader
- Providers need to identify their appropriate role, based on the context and the goals for the interaction
- Providers must analyze the communication setting and adapt their communication role to the patient or the situation and their goals

Ethics
- Requires using acceptable tactics and
  - Avoiding manipulating the patient or family member
  - Being honest and not trying to disguise information
  - Not insulting or demeaning the other person
  - Never making promises that can't be fulfilled
- Interpersonal relationships, trust, and collaboration depend on ethical behaviors by providers

INITIAL INTERACTION

Role play and/or analyze the following example:

Madison Leonard had just finished breast-feeding her newborn baby, Miles. She and her husband, Mark, were sitting in the hospital room when the provider entered the room.

Provider:	"I hear you're doing great."
Ms. Leonard:	"They said I'm going home today."
Provider:	"You'll feel better recovering at home. You had a normal vaginal delivery and you and your baby are doing well; and these days insurance companies only pay for a limited stay after a normal delivery."
Ms. Leonard:	"You're just throwing me out?"
Provider:	"No, we're not throwing you out. We've had you talk with the lactation counselor, and you're healing fine and your baby is doing well, so there's no reason for you to be here any longer."
Ms. Leonard:	"We pay money for insurance—why don't we get more benefits from it?"
Provider:	"I can't answer that; you'd need to talk with your insurance company. But this way you can have more family and friends over and share your joy with them."
Ms. Leonard:	"I have no joy; I'm terrified, and you're kicking me out the door."
Provider:	"I'm not kicking you out. You will do just fine at home and so will your baby."
Ms. Leonard:	"I'm going to complain to the head of this place; you don't care about me or my baby—you just wanted our money and now you want the bed."
Provider:	"That's not true. But I have no control over your insurance policy and what it covers."

Discussion Questions

1. How would you evaluate the communication in this scenario?

_____

_____

_____

_____

2. How has insurance and managed care impacted provider–patient communication? How are they affecting it?

_____

_____

_____

_____

3. Do you think it should be the provider's role to explain to patients about their speedy discharge? If so, why? If not, why not, and whose role should it be?

_____

_____

_____

_____

4. What do you think are the implications for the hospital–patient and provider–patient relationship, based on this interaction?

_____

_____

_____

_____

5. Do you think a patient, like the one in this scenario, is being sent home prematurely? If so, why? If not, why not?

_____

_____

_____

_____

6. Is there an ethical issue for the provider in this scenario? If so, what is it and why? If not, why not?

_____

_____

_____

_____

7. How might you have handled the situation differently? Be specific.

_____

_____

_____

_____

Interactive Activity

- Rewrite (individually or in a group) the interaction between the provider and the patient.
- Rewrite the conversation, and try to improve the communication effectiveness and interpersonal relationship between the provider and the patient.
- Compare your rewrite to the Alternate Interaction that follows.

Interaction Rewrite

_____

_____

_____

_____

_____

_____

_____

_____

_____

_____

_____

_____

_____

_____

_____

_____

_____

_____

_____

_____

_____

_____

_____

_____

_____

_____

_____

_____

_____

_____

_____

_____

_____

_____

_____

_____

_____

_____

_____

ALTERNATE INTERACTION

Provider:	"Hello, Mr. and Ms. Leonard. How are you doing today?"
Ms. Leonard:	"Well, we were just talking about the fact that we're both a little nervous about going home today. I know you told us several times that it's normal to go home two days after the baby is born, but I just don't know if we're ready."
Provider:	"Okay, let's talk about that. I certainly understand your concerns—you've got a new baby to take care of. So tell me what else is worrying you?"
Ms. Leonard:	"Well, I'm still a bit worried about the breast-feeding and all the dos and don'ts."
Provider:	"Good, I can totally understand. I know the lactation educator came by already, but I'll have her stop by again. We'll talk in detail about how to take care of your episiotomy wound; and the pediatrician is going to come by and talk to you about what to expect from the baby, and to tell you to call if you have any concerns."

Ms. Leonard: "Having things written down will help. And the breast-feeding person was great."

Provider: "Good, and you know we'll all be available by phone if you need us. We're not going away; we just won't be coming into your room every day."

Ms. Leonard: "That sounds good; I guess it's just scary with your first baby and not knowing what to do if something unexpected happens."

Provider: "You are so right. It's that fear of the unknown that really is the worst, and our job is to try and minimize or eliminate your unknown, by giving you information on what to do if something happens that you are not sure about. And then you'll have all our phone numbers in case you want to talk with us about something."

Ms. Leonard: "That makes me feel better; but it would sure be nice if I could stay another night or two."

Provider: "Well, you can call your insurance company and see if they'll approve it. Or if they won't, you can pay for the extra day out-of-pocket. But what you want to ask yourselves is—will it be any less worrisome if you leave tomorrow instead of today. For most new parents, it's the leaving the hospital that's the hard part, and whether it happens after two days or three days, doesn't usually make a lot of difference."

Ms. Leonard: "I think you're right. If I stay tonight, I'm still going to be worried about leaving tomorrow; so I guess if you all think it's safe for us to go, then we'll go. My mother had me at home, so she didn't even spend one night in a hospital."

Provider: "You are exactly right. I've been doing this for a lot of years, and I can tell you most people find leaving here hard, no matter how long it is after their delivery. We'll be available to help, and I know you'll do fine."

Ms. Leonard: "Thanks."

Follow-up Discussion

1. What are some of the key differences between the two scenarios?

_____

_____

_____

_____

2. How does the fact that the provider spoke with the patient several times before the delivery about the 48 hour's discharge help to reduce the "crisis" response of the first scenario?

_____

_____

_____

_____

3. What other verbal communication strategies did the provider utilize to minimize the patient's concerns?

_____

_____

_____

4. Would you have asked the lactation educator to make an extra stop to see the patient in order to reduce her concerns?

_____

_____

_____

_____

5. What is your opinion of offering the patient the option to call the insurance company for additional day and/or paying for it out-of-pocket?

_____

_____

_____

_____

Key Points

1. Communicating emotionally-charged information, like a great deal of health communication, can be enhanced by providers developing strategies for dealing with patients' or family-members' responses. Recognizing which contexts and situations, like postpartum discharges for new parents and post-Emergency Room visits for children with acute respiratory symptoms, can benefit from preplanned communication strategies, and will make it much easier for providers. Experienced providers have heard patients' and parents' concerns and questions, and such feedback should allow providers to develop responses that are empathic and patient-focused. Too often providers take patients' and/or parents' responses to third parties' decisions as

personal attacks, and risk communication deteriorating to verbal aggression. There-fore, instead of blaming things on third parties or refusing to be helpful, because it's not the provider's decision, she/he can determine a variety of alternatives, including enhanced verbal and written communication with the patient, to reduce the patient's or parent's fears and concerns.

2. Healthcare has become increasingly time-sensitive, and one approach is to decrease the time spent communicating with patients. However, as with many interpersonal relationships, when one partner in a conversation does not feel that she/he has been allowed to gather and/or share information, that person feels that the communica-tion was ineffective. Consequently, the ineffective communication frequently results in the need for additional meetings to try and clarify, reinforce, or provide additional information. Therefore, the thought that less communication saves time is frequently incorrect, and actually results in more time being required to effectively communi-cate. The more providers can try to answer patients' and/or family members' ques-tions and concerns sufficiently, the better their opportunity to decrease the need for follow-up communication later.

I ONLY HAVE NINE MINUTES OR SO
26

Before reading the interaction below, please consider the following topics:

Nonverbal communication
- Is observed and interpreted by the other person in a communication
- Includes behaviors linked to verbal messages
  - Tone of voice
  - Volume
  - Tempo
  - Rhythm
  - Resonance
- Includes the way people use space
  - Typically in the U.S. culture, the area closest to a person's body is reserved only for intimates

Listening
- Relies on a number of skills
  - Interpreting the whole message
    - Verbal
    - Nonverbal
  - Maintaining attention to the communicator
- Shows respect for the speaker
- Promotes an interpersonal relationship

Feedback
- Can be evaluated from a patient's or provider's
  - Facial expressions
    - Grimace or puzzled look
  - Eye behaviors
    - No eye contact may mean confusion
    - Eye contact to evaluate feedback and assure understanding
  - Gestures
    - Raised hand
  - Verbal messages
    - Questions
  - Body movements
    - Head nod or shaking
- Based on the other person's restatement of what was heard

INITIAL INTERACTION

Role play and/or analyze the following example:

Herbert Merriwether is a 56-year-old CEO of a small advertising company. He's had a cough and low-grade fever for the past couple of weeks. He doesn't smoke, and other than some malaise, he has no other symptoms.

Provider:	"Well, Mr. Merriwether, your examination is really unremarkable and your temperature is normal, so I think it's most likely bronchitis."
Mr. Merriwether:	"So you don't think I need a chest X-ray?"
Provider:	"No; you're not a smoker, you're not running any temperature here, you don't have any real sputum, and your lungs sound clear."
Mr. Merriwether:	"I guess I'm just concerned because it has been going on for a while now. Do you think an antibiotic would help?"
Provider:	"Again, since you're not a smoker, we generally don't prescribe antibiotics. These things are usually self-limited, and it's just a matter of waiting for the virus to run its course."

Mr. Merriwether:	"Well, I'm not going to be happy if I have to come see you again in a few days because it's not gone, or if I have to go see someone else while I'm traveling."
Provider:	"Oh, where are you traveling?"
Mr. Merriwether:	"Singapore, Hong Kong, and Beijing, this trip."
Provider:	"Wow, that's exciting! Why don't I do this?—I'll give you some nose spray to help with any nasal congestion and decrease a postnasal drip, and some cough medicine with a narcotic to help suppress your cough, especially at night. And I'll write you a script for some antibiotics that you can get filled if you are still having a problem before your trip. (The provider moves toward the door and grabs the knob.) How does that sound?"
Mr. Merriwether:	"I guess it sounds okay; but you sure seem to be in a hurry."
Provider:	"Well, I want to get you better, but managed care says I have only nine minutes or so per patient to meet my quota, so I'm just trying to get everyone seen. Have a good trip."

Discussion Questions

1. How would you evaluate the communication in this scenario?

2. Do you think managed care or the provider is predominantly impacting this provider–patient relationship and communication?

3. How do you think the provider's communication in this scenario may have affected the information exchange and the patient's diagnosis and treatment?

4. Do you think, based on the provider's explanation to the patient, that the diagnosis and treatment is reasonable? If so, why? If not, why not?

_____

_____

_____

_____

_____

5. What information from the patient's statement needed some further exploration by the provider?

_____

_____

_____

6. How do you think the provider's need to meet his/her patient quota for the day impacted this interaction, data-gathering, and relationship-building?

_____

_____

_____

_____

7. How do you think the provider's nonverbal communication of asking a question and grabbing the door knob affected the patient's perception of the provider, the relationship, and the provider's recommendations?

_____

_____

_____

_____

_____

_____

Interactive Activity

- Rewrite (individually or in a group) the interaction between the provider and the patient.
- Rewrite the conversation, and try to improve the communication effectiveness, data-gathering, and interpersonal relationship between the provider and the patient.
- Compare your rewrite to the Alternate Interaction that follows.

Interaction Rewrite

ALTERNATE INTERACTION

The provider and Mr. Merriwether are in an examination room. The provider is making eye contact, while seated on a rolling chair next to the patient, who is dressed and sitting in a chair.

Provider:	"Mr. Merriwether, I haven't really found any bacterial cause for your cough. You don't have a fever here; did you take any medicine earlier today?"
Mr. Merriwether:	"Oh yeah, I forgot, I did take a couple of Ibuprofen about two hours ago."
Provider:	"That explains the lack of fever. But your lungs sound good, your throat looks fine, and your sinuses are nontender. Any blood in your sputum?"
Mr. Merriwether:	"No blood; just clear stuff."
Provider:	"How about traveling—have you traveled very much lately?"
Mr. Merriwether:	"Are you kidding? That's all I do. I've been to India, Hong Kong, and Tokyo, all in the last six months, and I'm getting ready to go to Singapore, Hong Kong, and Beijing in two weeks—that's why I need to get this cleared up."
Provider:	"Okay, so you've been traveling a lot. Have you ever had a Purified Protein Derivative (PPD)—a TB test on your arm?"
Mr. Merriwether:	"No, I don't remember that. You think I've got TB?"
Provider:	"I don't know, but it would explain your symptoms, and some of the countries you've been traveling to have a higher incidence of TB. Since you have symptoms, I'm going to do a chest X-ray and plant a TB test on your arm. Then I'm going to call an infectious disease specialist and get you an appointment."
Mr. Merriwether:	"Okay, no problem. But what happens if I've got it?"
Provider:	"Well, if your TB test is positive, they'll want to check your sputum and start you on Isonaizid (INH)—the medicine to treat TB."
Mr. Merriwether:	"Can I travel?"
Provider:	"I'll let you talk about that with Dr. Pavlis, but usually they make you wear a mask until your sputum returns to normal."
Mr. Merriwether:	"You're scaring me a little."
Provider:	"I don't want to scare you; I just want to let you know what I know, and how we're going to do more tests to try and figure out what is causing your symptoms."
Mr. Merriwether:	"Okay, but I really need to go to Asia in a couple of weeks."
Provider:	"I would think that might be possible, but again, Dr. Pavlis will talk with you about all that once all the tests are done. But remember, you don't

have any blood in your sputum, and it's only been two weeks of symptoms, so this could all be related to a virus. Now, let me go get you an
appointment and we'll get the chest X-ray and plant the TB test on your
arm. And I'm going to give you some handouts on TB, so you can do
some reading. Any more questions?"

Mr. Merriwether: "Not right now; but I'm sure I'll have more after I read the handouts."

Provider: (Stands up.) "I'm sure you will have questions, and that's why it will be
good if you can read the handouts before you see Dr. Pavlis, so she can
answer them. But you can always call me. Now let's get these tests done,
and I'll get the appointment set up; and I'm going to have them fit you
for a mask because, until we know what this is for sure, it's safest to protect those you are around—just in case it is TB."

Mr. Merriwether: "A mask, wow, this is too weird, but let's do it. I don't want to give
anyone else something I've got."

Provider: (Extends a hand to shake the patient's hand.) "We'll get this all figured out,
but in the meantime, we just want to be sure we don't spread anything."

Follow-up Discussion

1. What are some of the key differences between the two scenarios?

2. How did the interaction in the second scenario alter the diagnosis and treatment plan?

3. How did the provider's communication of next steps help to move the process for-
ward and enhance the provider–patient relationship?

4. Why would the provider–patient relationship in this particular scenario be very important?

_____

_____

_____

_____

5. Would you offer to accept calls from the patient with questions, even after you've referred him to a specialist? If so, what are some of the potential issues that could arise? If not, why not?

_____

_____

_____

_____

_____

_____

Key Points

1. While it is true that managed care and other factors have altered the time that some providers can routinely spend with patients, an effective exchange of information must occur. When providers' and patients' communication are impacted in a way that limits the discussion, investigation, and analysis of the patient's complaints or problems, an accurate diagnosis and successful outcome may not be possible.

2. Providers need to remember that nonverbal behaviors often communicate more to patients than verbal communication. For example, asking a question with a hand on the door knob communicates the provider's interest in leaving and lack of interest in the patient's answer to the question. Be aware of your nonverbal cues, and make sure they match your intended communication if you want to minimize confusion and decrease a patient's negative responses.

3. Because of the nature of the interaction, patients often forget, or fail to provide all the information needed to make a diagnosis and accurately assess the problem. Therefore, providers have to be aware of the important role that listening and feedback play in obtaining the information needed to evaluate the patient's condition. By letting the patient tell his/her story and then providing feedback via questions to clarify or expand the details, the provider can greatly enhance the breadth and depth of the information obtained.

Why Don't You Tell Me About It?
27

Before reading the interaction below, please consider the following topics:

Family communication
- Providers frequently need to communicate with patients' family members
- Under HIPAA, adult patients must give formal permission for their health status or information to be communicated to anyone
  - Family members may expect to be informed automatically

Trust
- Key to collaboration and successful goal-attainment
- Depends on each communicator believing she/he can rely on the other
- In groups, everyone is working for the best interest of the group and not for the individual
- Results from effective interpersonal communication

Health Literacy
- Affects health outcomes
- Typically refers to
  - Cultural knowledge
  - Verbal skills
  - Writing and reading skills
- Relies on the provider's assessment of the patient's literacy level

INITIAL INTERACTION

Role play and/or analyze the following example:

Miles Addison is a 6-year-old boy, who cut his finger and is in an Urgent Care Center with his mother. The provider enters the room as Miles starts to cry.

Provider: "Hi. What are you crying about; I haven't even touched you."

Ms. Addison: "He was playing with some glass and he cut his finger."

Provider: "Okay, so let's take a peek."

Ms. Addison: "Is it going to need stitches?"

Miles: "What are stitches?"

Provider: "Yeah, see how it gapes open when he bends it."

Miles: "What are stitches?"

Provider: "Okay, so here's what's going to happen Ms. Addison: we'll get set up here, and they'll put some special medicine on a gauze pad that he can hold on his finger for 15 minutes or so, which will make it partially numb; then we'll get it fixed up."

Ms. Addison: "Do we need a plastic surgeon?"

Provider: "That's up to you; if you want, we can call one, but since this isn't on his face or very big, they may not come out for it. And I'm sure he wouldn't be here for at least an hour or two."

Miles: "What are stitches?"

Ms. Addison: "Wait just a minute, Miles. So what would you do?"

Provider: "Well, I sew these up every day; so if it were my son, I'd have me close it. But you can do whatever you want."

Ms. Addison: "Okay, but is it going to hurt?"

Provider: "Only for a few seconds, then he won't feel it anymore."

Miles: "I want to feel it." (Miles starts crying again.)

Discussion Questions

1. How would you evaluate the communication in this scenario?

    _____
    _____
    _____
    _____

2. How would you assess the provider's verbal and nonverbal communication with the mom, and with Miles?

    _____
    _____
    _____
    _____
    _____

3. Would you have communicated differently with Miles? If so, why? If not, why not?

    _____
    _____
    _____
    _____

4. With a 6-year-old patient, how do you change your communication strategy, especially when dealing with a problem that will require you to cause the patient some pain and require his/her cooperation?

    _____
    _____
    _____
    _____

5. Do you think suturing Miles' finger will be impacted by the lack of provider–patient communication? If so, why and how? If not, why not?

    _____
    _____
    _____
    _____

Interactive Activity

- Rewrite (individually or in a group) the interaction between the provider and the patient and parent of the patient.
- Rewrite the conversation, and try to improve the communication effectiveness and information-sharing between the provider and the patient.
- Compare your rewrite to the Alternate Interaction that follows.

Interaction Rewrite

_____

_____

_____

_____

_____

_____

_____

_____

_____

_____

_____

_____

_____

_____

_____

ALTERNATE INTERACTION

Insert your name and/or profession in the appropriate blanks below.

The provider knocks on the door, enters the examination room, and goes directly to Miles and shakes his hand.

Provider:	"Hi, Miles. My name is _____, and I'm a ____. I hear you hurt your finger."
Ms. Addison:	"He was playing. . . ."
Provider:	"I'm sorry to interrupt, but I'd like to talk to Miles; then we can talk if we need to. Okay Miles, now you tell me what happened."
Miles:	"I fell on the playground and glass cut my finger."
Provider:	"That's not very nice of that glass."
Miles:	"Are you going to give me a shot?"
Provider:	"Well, let's see your finger; can you move it for me?"

Miles:	"Like that?"
Provider:	"Does it hurt?"
Miles:	"No."
Provider:	"I thought you might say that. Okay, so here's the deal, Miles: when you move your finger, see how the cut gets bigger?"
Miles:	"Yeah."
Provider:	"That means it will be hard for it to heal without our help. So I need to fix it."
Miles:	"How do you do that?"
Provider:	"We'll put some medicine on top of your finger and it will make your finger feel like it's asleep. Then we'll put some medicine in around your cut, and we'll fix it so you can go home."
Miles:	"So no shots?"
Provider:	"No shots like you get in your arm up here. But after your finger feels like it's asleep, we'll put some more medicine in it and that might sting for a minute or so, but then it won't hurt any more. Can you be brave and help me fix your finger?"
Miles:	"I guess so. Can Mom stay?"
Provider:	"You bet she can. We'll put a chair right next to the bed for her, and she can hold your other hand. Ms. Addison, do you have any questions?"
Ms. Addison:	"No; will he be able to go to swim class?"
Provider:	"You bet. He'll need to keep it dry for 24 hours, and then he can go into the pool or the shower. He had his tetanus shot before he went to school?"
Ms. Addison:	"Yes, he's had them all."
Provider:	"Great! So he won't need that. Okay, Miles, any questions before I go?"
Miles:	"Will you be back?"
Provider:	"Yes, we'll put that medicine on a little pad and lay it on your cut. Can you hold it on there for me?"
Miles:	"Yes."
Provider:	"Okay, so I'll be back in a little bit."

Follow-up Discussion

1. What are some of the key differences between the two scenarios?

_____

_____

_____

_____

2. How comfortable are you talking with children about their illnesses or injuries? If so, why. If not, why not?

_____

_____

_____

_____

3. How did the provider's nonverbal and verbal communication change the patient's and his mother's responses to the interaction? Why do you think that happened?

_____

_____

_____

_____

_____

_____

4. Do you think the child's trust of the provider is enhanced more in the first or the second interaction?

_____

_____

_____

_____

5. How do you keep pediatric patient interactions from being third-party communication, with the patient being a nonperson in the room?

_____

_____

_____

_____

Key Points

1. Pediatric patients may not be able to give a complete history, but they usually respond well to being included in the interaction. The more a provider can build a relationship with a pediatric patient, the easier it will be to gain his/her cooperation and trust.

2. Even though some procedures cause pain, the more information a provider can supply to patients, especially pediatric patients, the better the chance of reducing some of their fears. Because communication is continuous, pediatric patients remember especially the pain previously caused by providers and immunizations, and

often it's the fear of what they remember that impacts their abilities to understand their present situation. Therefore, the more a provider can try to explain the current situation, how it differs from previous ones, what will happen, and what will hurt and what won't, the greater the likelihood that the patient will cooperate and have a more positive response.

3. Communicating with pediatric patients and their parents requires providers to use various levels of health literacy, and to try and develop an interpersonal relationship with each interactant. It's always important to remember that just because a patient is very young, she/he still can communicate, and they can choose to cooperate and participate or to make the process much more difficult for everyone. A little time spent communicating with pediatric patients and parents alike will result in a much greater opportunity for trust and a more rewarding outcome.

V

CULTURE
AND
HEALTH
COMMUNICATION

We Just Need to Get Through the Chemo

28

Before reading the interaction below, please consider the following topics:

End-of-life communication
- Too often not effectively utilized by providers
  - Discussions of advanced care directives or living wills are important conversations that need to occur between providers and older and/or at-risk patients
- Providers need to conceptualize end-of-life communication, not as a depressing or hopeless conversation, but as empowering the patient to take control of his/her situation
  - Should include a discussion of the patient's values, so that the provider can honor the patient's wishes

Family communication
- Family communication needs to be about more than the patient only—also about the caregiver(s)
- Caregivers are influenced by the patients with whom they interact
  - The more problems a patient has, the more work will likely result for the caregiver
  - Family members need to assess patients' complaints, especially for those with terminal illnesses, and help them make decisions about their care, who to contact, and when
- Too often family members, as caregivers, don't communicate their own issues to providers, and their health suffers

INITIAL INTERACTION
Role play and/or analyze the following example:

Nicholas Hunt is waiting in the provider's examination room. Mr. Hunt is a 73-year-old male, who was recently diagnosed with a grade IV astrocytoma. He's in the office to discuss his treatment options. The provider enters the examination room and proceeds to a computer on wheels that is next to the examination table.

Provider: "Hi, Mr. Hunt. Give me just a minute to pull up your chart on the computer."

Mr. Hunt: "Okay."

Provider: "So as we discussed the other day, the biopsy showed it was an astrocytoma. And it's fairly advanced, so I think we need to get pretty aggressive here."

Mr. Hunt: "What's that mean?"

Provider: "Well, I'm recommending we do radiation and chemotherapy, and see if we can shrink this thing down."

Mr. Hunt: "Does that work?"

Provider: "We've had some success, but everyone is different, and you may have a tumor that responds very well to one or both modalities."

Mr. Hunt: "What's a modality?"

Provider: "You know—chemo. or radiation. Now I'd like to get you set up to go over to meet up with the radiation folks, so they can get you all scheduled and mapped out."

Mr. Hunt: "Mapped out?"

Provider: "They have to figure out the best spot to direct the beam, and they'll want to do some tests to be sure they have the best path for the radiation to travel."

Mr. Hunt: "Is that going to hurt?"

Provider: "No, it won't, and they'll be able to answer all your questions over there. So let me type this in, and I'll give them a call and get you over there."

Mr. Hunt: "So how long do I have to do this for?"

Provider: "Hold on, I can't type and talk to you. Just let me finish your record here, and then I'll get you on your way."

Discussion Questions

1. How would you evaluate the communication in this scenario?

   _____

   _____

   _____

   _____

2. How would you assess the provider's nonverbal communication?

   _____

   _____

   _____

   _____

   _____

3. What is your opinion of having a computer in the examination room and typing the record during the patient's visit?

   _____

   _____

   _____

4. Since this is an older gentleman, with a brain tumor, do you think the provider should have requested that the patient bring a family member or patient advocate with him to the interaction? If so, why? If not, why not?

   _____

   _____

   _____

   _____

5. What information, based on the scenario, do you think is missing from this communication, and why do you think the provider didn't discuss it?

   _____

   _____

   _____

   _____

6. In terms of leadership communication (directing the patient's treatment), would you classify the provider's style as authoritarian or participatory?

_____

_____

_____

_____

7. There is no discussion by the provider of the patient's prognosis. Why do you think that is avoided? Do you agree with this approach? If so, why? If not, why not?

_____

_____

_____

_____

_____

Interactive Activity

- Rewrite (individually or in a group) the interaction between the provider and the patient.
- Create a conversation, and try to improve the communication effectiveness and information-sharing between the provider and the patient.
- Compare your rewrite to the Alternate Interaction that follows.

Interaction Rewrite

_____

_____

_____

_____

_____

_____

_____

_____

_____

_____

_____

_____

ALTERNATE INTERACTION

Mr. Hunt and his daughter, Julia Feliciano, are in the provider's office. The three of them are seated around a small table.

Provider:	"Hello, Mr. Hunt, and it's Ms. Feliciano, isn't it?"
Ms. Feliciano:	"It is."
Mr. Hunt:	"Hi, how are you?"
Provider:	"I'm fine, and thanks for asking. But more importantly, how are you doing?"
Mr. Hunt:	"My head hurts sometimes, but no more seizures."
Provider:	"I'm sorry about the headaches, but I'm really glad about the seizures."
Mr. Hunt:	"Me, too. So now what?"
Provider:	"Well, I asked you and Julia to come in today because we need to make some decisions about what to do now that we have some answers."
Mr. Hunt:	"I like answers."
Provider:	"As we talked about after the biopsy, you have a very serious brain tumor and that's what caused your seizures and headaches. So now we need to talk about what happens next. Have you had a chance to read over the information I printed out for you?"
Mr. Hunt:	"I read it, but I needed to do it in small amounts, because reading for too long makes my head hurt."
Provider:	"And Ms. Feliciano, did you get to read any of it?"
Ms. Feliciano:	"I read it. It sounds like it can make him very sick, and it doesn't seem to do a lot of good."
Provider:	"Well, with tumors like the one your dad has, we don't have a lot of long-term success; but some of these tumors respond to radiation, and there are not a lot of bad side effects."
Mr. Hunt:	"So you're recommending radiation?"
Provider:	"I think we should start by you talking to the radiation specialists, and see what they have to say and what they think will be the risks and rewards of having treatment."
Mr. Hunt:	"Sounds like my golf game—go for the green or lay up."
Provider:	"That's a good analogy. I play a little golf myself. What you need to decide is how much discomfort you are willing to put up with to try and get some reduction in the size of the tumor."
Ms. Feliciano:	"So we're not talking cure."

Provider: "No, these types of tumors are almost never cured. The best we can do is to shrink it as much as possible and slow its growth. But what we don't want is for the treatment to cause more discomfort than the tumor."

Mr. Hunt: "So it's going to kill me."

Provider: "Well, nothing is 100% in medicine, but usually these tumors can only be slowed down, not stopped. So what we're trying to do is give you the best quality of life we can for however long you have, and maybe you can play golf for a while longer."

Mr. Hunt: "I'd like that, and to spend time with Julia and my grandkids."

Provider: "That makes good sense to me. So what I'd like you to do is go talk to the radiation oncologist, and get as much information and ask as many questions as you can. Then you and Julia can discuss the pros and cons of having radiation. Once you decide, then we'll discuss chemo, but I'd like you to decide about the radiation first."

Mr. Hunt: "So how long do I have?"

Provider: "I don't know the answer to that; it really depends on what treatments you choose and how your tumor responds. But if you decide not to treat it, you probably have less than a year and it could be even shorter. I know this is very difficult and hard to understand all at once, so I'm going to call you tomorrow to see if you have any questions, or if you want to go over some of this again."

Mr. Hunt: "Thanks, it's really a bit much."

Provider: "I know it is, and I want you to call me with any questions. I also want to encourage you to take some time in the next few days to get your end-of-life decisions made. It's something that will make it easier for you and for your family. Make sure your will is in order, and then decide whether you want to have a living will."

Mr. Hunt: "That's done; my wife and I got our wills done before she died, and both of us did a living will. I don't want to be on a machine if I'm not coming back. And neither did she, and that made it easier when she had the stroke and couldn't talk."

Follow-up Discussion

1. What are some of the key differences between the two scenarios?

_____

_____

_____

_____

2. How comfortable are you talking with patients and their families about end-of-life issues? Why do you feel that way?

_____

_____

_____

_____

3. Do you agree that patients who are facing major treatment decisions, and who have potentially terminal illnesses, should be discussing end-of-life and quality-of-life issues with the provider as well? If so, why? If not, why not?

_____

_____

_____

_____

_____

_____

4. How does the provider, in this scenario versus the first one, use nonverbal and verbal communication to enhance the relationship-building and information-exchange?

_____

_____

_____

_____

5. How does culture, the patient, and his family's values and beliefs, potentially impact the decision-making here, and how can a provider communicate appropriately and empower the patient?

_____

_____

_____

_____

_____

Key Points

1. There are many types of cultures and co-cultures. For example, the interactants in this scenario are all from the same American culture, but the patient is from a co-culture (older adult males), the patient and his daughter are from a co-culture (their family), and the provider is from a variety of co-cultures—different in some ways and similar in others to that of the patient. Because various cultures and co-cultures have different values and beliefs, it's important for providers not to try and impose their values and beliefs on others. At the same time, it's important to help patients, especially those with terminal illnesses, to understand the reality of the situation, and to help them prepare for the end of their lives. Being a healthcare provider and an effective communicator requires that not only the biological, but also the psychological and sociological aspects of treating an illness be discussed. In addition, wills and living wills are very important end-of-life decisions from both psychological and sociological perspectives.

2. For a critically difficult interaction, like discussions of a terminal illness, patients need support to retain information, ask questions, and make decisions. It's often very helpful for a person to have a family member or friend participate in the discussion. The important communication role of a patient advocate, as a support person in highly emotional communication healthcare settings, cannot be overstated.

3. Human beings want hope, but we also need factual information in order to make empowered decisions. For terminally ill patients, medical information should also include a discussion of end-of-life issues that need to be addressed. Patients may not be able to make such decisions at the moment they are discussed. However, a provider who recognizes the emotions of the moment will more likely present the information and follow-up on it a day or two later, after the patient has had a chance to assimilate all the details, discuss them with family or friends, and prepare questions or arrive at a decision.

No Hablo Español

29

Before reading the interaction below, please consider the following topics:

Intercultural communication
- Includes the sharing of information between individuals who are culturally different
  - People belong to a culture
    - An ethnic group
  - Most people belong to several different co-cultures
    - Male, female
    - Teenager, adult, student
    - Daughter, son
    - Professional, nonprofessional
- Providers need to understand their patients' cultural backgrounds in order to communicate effectively
  - Some patients may not share the same language or symbols as the provider
  - Other patients may have different values or beliefs that prevent them from actively participating in decision-making

Information-sharing
- A sender has to use symbols to put a thought or idea into a message
- A receiver of the message has to be able to interpret the symbols and derive the sender's idea or thought
- For information-sharing to occur, both the sender and receiver of messages have to share the same symbols
- Collaborative communication and decision-making rely on effective information-sharing

INITIAL INTERACTION

Role play and/or analyze the following example:

Manuel Orontes is 35-year-old Hispanic male, who is in the Fast Track area of an Emergency Department, complaining of a sore throat. His vital signs (temperature, pulse, respiration rate, pulse oximeter, and blood pressure) are all normal. The provider enters the room and the patient is looking out the window.

Provider:	"Hello. Mr. Orontes?"
Mr. Orontes:	"Hola! ¿Habla Español?"
Provider:	"Not really. Family?"
Mr. Orontes:	"No."
Provider:	"Great. Dolor?"
Mr. Orontes:	"Si." (He points to his throat.)
Provider:	"¿Calor?"
Mr. Orontes:	"No."
Provider:	"Cough?" (Provider mimics a cough.)
Mr. Orontes:	"No. Dolor aqui." (He points to his throat.)
Provider:	"¿Cuantos dias?"
Mr. Orontes:	"Tres dias."
Provider:	"Okay, three days of a sore throat without fever or cough. I'm going to look in your mouth. Abre la boca!"
Mr. Orontes:	"Ahh."
Provider:	"Bueno, no mas rojo. Virus, ¿comprende?"
Mr. Orontes:	"¡Dolor!"

Discussion Questions

1. How would you evaluate the communication in this scenario?

_____

_____

_____

_____

2. How does the provider's attempt to communicate with the patient in Spanish enhance or hinder the information-exchange and the provider–patient relationship?

_____

_____

_____

_____

3. How do you perceive the diagnostic evaluation of this patient's visit?

_____

_____

_____

4. How do the cultural differences and societal realities impact this scenario, and how would you have handled it differently?

_____

_____

_____

_____

_____

5. What information, based on the scenario, do you think is missing from this communication?

_____

_____

_____

_____

6. Assuming the provider did a Rapid Strep. Test and it was negative, are you comfortable with the "virus" diagnosis? If so, why? If not, why not?

_____

_____

_____

7. As the U.S. population continues to evolve, cultural differences beyond language become obvious. Can you discuss some of these differences related to this scenario and the problems they present for information-exchange between providers and patients?

_____

_____

_____

_____

Interactive Activity

- Rewrite (individually or in a group) the interaction between the provider and the patient.
- Rewrite the conversation, and try to improve the communication effectiveness and information-sharing between the provider and the patient.
- Compare your rewrite to the Alternate Interaction that follows.

Interaction Rewrite

_____

_____

_____

_____

_____

_____

_____

_____

_____

_____

_____

_____

_____

_____

_____

_____

_____

_____

_____

_____

_____

_____

_____

_____

_____

_____

_____
_____
_____
_____
_____
_____
_____
_____
_____
_____
_____
_____
_____
_____
_____

ALTERNATE INTERACTION

The provider enters the patient's room with a telephone that has two headsets.

Provider:	"¡Hola!"
Mr. Orontes:	"¡Hola!"
Provider:	"¿Ingles?"
Mr. Orontes:	"No. ¿Habla Español?"
Provider:	"No, muy poquito Español. Un momento, por favor." (The provider dials a number on the multi-headset phone.)
Voice-on-phone:	"This is language translator number 20167. Do you need English to Spanish translation?"
Provider:	"Yes. The patient is Manuel."

Voice-on-phone:	"I'll be happy to translate for you, and I'll repeat exactly what each of you says."
Provider:	"Great. Please ask him what's bothering him?"
Voice-on-phone:	"He says about three days ago he was having lunch and he got a pain in his throat, and it's been hurting him ever since."
Provider:	"What was he eating?"
Voice-on-phone:	"He says a chicken sandwich."
Provider:	"Anything else bothering him besides the pain?"
Voice-on-phone:	"He says that he can't eat; it feels like something is stuck, and it hurts?"
Provider:	"Has he vomited?"
Voice-on-phone:	"No, but he says he hasn't eaten any food, because he's afraid he'll choke or vomit, or it will hurt."
Provider:	"Ask him if he's had any drooling?"
Voice-on-phone:	"He doesn't think so."
Provider:	"Okay. Please tell him I understand he was eating a chicken sandwich three days ago, felt something in his throat, and since then has had pain and trouble swallowing. And he's not eating because he's afraid of choking."
Voice-on-phone:	"He says yes."
Provider:	"Tell him I'm going to examine his throat and listen to his lungs and heart, and then we're going to do some tests. Please let him know that I think he might have a chicken bone lodged in his throat or in his esophagus—the food pipe that goes to his stomach. If the tests show that he does, we'll have a specialist get it out. If not, then it's just some irritation, and we'll get him some medicine for that."
Voice-on-phone:	"He wants to know if he has to have surgery."
Provider:	"No; usually they can get a bone out, if he has one, with a scope that goes into his throat."
Voice-on-phone:	"He's worried about work; he needs to make money to send back home."
Provider:	"Tell him I understand. This should not keep him from working, except maybe a day or two, but he needs to get it fixed or it will cause him more problems and more missed work."
Mr. Orontes:	"¡Gracias!"
Provider:	"Please tell him I'm happy to help, and he needs to be patient while I examine him and we schedule the test, but we should get some answers soon. We'll need to call you back at that time, okay?"
Voice-on-phone:	"I'll tell him, and we'll be happy to help whenever you need us."

Follow-up Discussion

1. What are some of the key differences between the two scenarios?

   _____

   _____

   _____

   _____

2. Have you ever used a telephone translator? If so, how did you find the communication experience? If not, what are some of the advantages and disadvantages for the provider and the patient?

   _____

   _____

   _____

   _____

3. From a cultural perspective, how do you think you would feel if you were a patient in another country and the provider didn't speak your language or share your cultural beliefs? How would that affect your perception of the diagnosis?

   _____

   _____

   _____

   _____

4. What are the key interpersonal communication differences between the first and the alternate interaction?

   _____

   _____

5. What might be some reason(s) why this patient did not bring family or friends with him to the Emergency Department? How might that decision impact the outcome?

   _____

   _____

   _____

   _____

Key Points

1. Effective health communication, the exchange of information, and building and maintaining of interpersonal relationships are critical to successful provider–patient interactions and outcomes. The basis for this communication exchange is the use, by both communicators, of shared symbols. These symbols include both verbal symbols (language) and nonverbal symbols (cues). Without a shared understanding of a sender's or receiver's symbols, effective communication cannot be accomplished. In addition to language barriers, cultural differences in beliefs and values can also impact the provider–patient setting. For example, some cultures do not want to include family and friends in their discussions about their health, while other cultures find it important to share such emotional experiences with family and/or friends. It's important for providers to understand that cultural differences impact the communication exchange in many ways.

2. While it may be possible to minimally communicate with a person using a language that a provider does not fully comprehend or speak, generally that is not sufficient to exchange the information needed for an accurate diagnosis and appropriate treatment plan. Veterinary medicine requires diagnosis and treatment without verbal communication with the patient. The major advantage that verbal communication provides to human healthcare is lost with patients and providers who do not speak the same language (share the same symbols). In order to benefit from this shared language, however, providers need to find ways to make the interaction truly a shared experience. Telephone translators, or the use of family members or friends who are approved by the patient, can be enormously helpful to both patients and providers in such a setting. However, with Health Insurance Portability and Accountability Act (HIPAA) rules, strangers and nonclinical hospital or office personnel cannot be drafted to translate. Providers must walk a fine line of knowing enough about a culture's language, values, and beliefs to communicate effectively with a patient, or they must find a legally acceptable translator to help with the accurate exchange of information. In doing so, providers will be helping to build a relationship across cultures.

HEALTH INSURANCE PORTABILITY AND ACCOUNTABILITY ACT (HIPAA)
30

Before reading the interaction below, please consider the following topics:

Organizational communication
- Providers work under corporate, state, and federal policies
- Organizations communicate policies to providers through a variety of formats
  - Memos
  - Internet
  - Policy and procedure manuals
  - E-mail
- Providers are responsible for knowing the various organizations' policies and following them
  - HIPAA is a federal government regulation
  - Individual organizations have policies related to how HIPAA is to be followed by providers and employees

Family communication
- Families are a co-culture
  - Like other co-cultures, families have their own unique attributes and communication styles
  - Some families like to share everything
  - Some families have members who want their independence
- Providers have to know HIPAA regulations as well as patients' desires regarding family communication
- An adult patient's requests regarding family communication must take precedence over a family's desire for information

INITIAL INTERACTION
Role play and/or analyze the following example:

Pamela Morton is the mother of Celia Morton, a 19-year-old college student, who was taken to an Emergency Department near the university where she is a sophomore. Ms. Morton is calling from her home 2,000 miles away. She is speaking with a healthcare provider at the Emergency Department about her daughter.

Provider:	"Hello."
Ms. Morton:	"I'm trying to find out about my daughter, Celia. The campus police called and said she was taken to the ER."
Provider:	"I understand, but under HIPAA regulations, I can't tell you anything about her, except that she is here."
Ms. Morton:	"I'm her mother."
Provider:	"I understand, but unfortunately, there's no way for me to confirm that and even if I could, she's an adult and has to give permission for us to talk to anyone."
Ms. Morton:	"Then go ask her!"
Provider:	"I can't do that."
Ms. Morton:	"Then let me talk to someone who's in charge."
Provider:	"This is a federal regulation. It has nothing to do with being in charge. As soon as she can complete the HIPAA release form, we'll be in touch."
Ms. Morton:	"What's wrong with her that she can't complete a form?"
Provider:	"I can't discuss her condition. We'll be in touch when we have her permission."
Ms. Morton:	"This is wrong; I'm 2,000 miles away!"
Provider:	"I'm sorry; I don't make federal policies. If you give me your phone number, I'll call as soon as I get her permission."
Ms. Morton:	"This is unfair. I'm going to be sitting here, scared to death, until you call."
Provider:	"I'll call you back just as soon as I get her permission."

Discussion Questions

1. How would you evaluate the communication in this scenario?

   _____

   _____

   _____

   _____

2. How does the culture of the Emergency Department add to the communication problems in this scenario?

    _____

    _____

    _____

    _____

    _____

3. If you were the Emergency Department provider, how would you have handled this interaction—in the same way or differently, and why?

    _____

    _____

    _____

    _____

    _____

4. What are some of the cultural values and beliefs of a family that might conflict with the cultural values and beliefs of an Emergency Department?

    _____

    _____

    _____

    _____

    _____

5. How do you reconcile the differences between organizational policies and people's needs or requests for information?

    _____

    _____

    _____

    _____

    _____

Interactive Activity

- Rewrite (individually or in a group) the interaction between the provider and the patient's family member.
- Rewrite the conversation, and try to improve the communication effectiveness and information-sharing between the provider and the patient's mother.
- Compare your rewrite to the Alternate Interaction that follows.

Interaction Rewrite

ALTERNATE INTERACTION
Insert your name and/or profession in the appropriate blanks below.

The provider answers the phone in the Emergency Department.

Provider: "Hello. This is _____; I'm a _____."

Ms. Morton: "Hi. This is Celia Morton's mother, and I just got a call from the campus police that my daughter was brought in there. I need to know what's going on and they wouldn't tell me."

Provider: "I'm sorry to say you're not going to be much happier with me."

Ms. Morton: "What's going on? Why all the secrecy."

Provider: "I don't think I would categorize it as secrecy; but several years ago the government created HIPAA regulations, and since that time we need a patient's permission to talk with anyone about his or her condition, disposition, or treatment."

Ms. Morton: "That's the most stupid thing I've ever heard of. I'm her mom!"

Provider: "I know you say that, but I have no way to prove that and even if I could, I would still need your daughter's consent."

Ms. Morton: "So how long am I going to have to wait—I'm scared to death!"

Provider: "I understand it must be very scary. Let me try to go get her permission and I'll call you back just as soon as possible."

Ms. Morton: "Oh, thank you so much; I'm so worried and I can't believe I don't know how she is."

Provider: "I'll be in touch."
(Some time later.)

Ms. Morton: "Hello. This is Pam Morton."

Provider: "Hi. This is _____, the _____ in the Emergency Department."

Ms. Morton: "Oh, thank God; I thought you'd never call back!"

Provider: "Well, part of the problem was I had to wait until Celia sobered up in order to get her permission."

Ms. Morton: "She's drunk?"

Provider: "She was when she came in. Apparently she'd been to a party and drank until she blacked out, and then her friends called the campus police and they called an ambulance."

Ms. Morton: "I didn't even know she drank."

Provider:	"Well, we will certainly discuss her drinking and the risks with her before she leaves, and we'll be giving her the name of a psychologist to see about this problem."
Ms. Morton:	"You think she has a drinking problem?"
Provider:	"Her blood alcohol level was over twice the normal limit. And she was trying to pass out, according to her friends—so we do think she has a drinking problem and a much distorted sense of what her risks are, drinking like she did."
Ms. Morton:	"Is she okay?"
Provider:	"She's doing fine; she's been vomiting and we're giving her IV fluids, so she's getting better, and she's starting to understand what happened and how many people she's scared."
Ms. Morton:	"I don't know whether to be angry with her or feel sorry for her."
Provider:	"She's obviously a bright young woman, but she's made some poor decisions. However, she's on the mend. Would you like me to let you talk with her?"
Ms. Morton:	"Does she want to talk with me?"
Provider:	"She does, but she's worried you're going to be mad at her."
Ms. Morton:	"I don't think now's the time for that, do you?"
Provider:	"I agree. You can have a heart-to-heart conversation with her later."
Ms. Morton:	"I think you're right. Thanks."
Provider:	"I'll transfer you to her. Best of luck, and I'm glad everything worked out."

Follow-up Discussion

1. What are some of the key differences between the two scenarios?

2. What are your perceptions of the way the provider communicated in the alternate scenario, from a HIPAA perspective and from a relationship-building perspective?

3. From a cultural perspective, how do you think the provider managed the intercultural issues related to the hospital organization's culture and the family's culture?

_____

_____

_____

4. What are the key interpersonal communication differences between the first and the alternate interaction?

_____

_____

_____

5. Discuss how the health provider's role and the communication role, in this scenario, are linked by the need to overcome the difficulties presented by HIPAA in such a setting? Be specific, and discuss why you feel the way you do?

_____

_____

_____

_____

Key Points

1. While there are policy and communication issues that appear to be polar opposites, as with many things, compromise and understanding can help overcome such obstacles and improve information-sharing and outcomes. The provider had to follow the organization's and HIPAA's policies regarding communication. Therefore, the provider could have said "no" and ended the conversation with the parent. By trying to empathize with the mother's situation and still get the patient's permission, the provider illustrated her/his professionalism and willingness to assist both the patient and the parent.

2. The culture of the Emergency Department usually necessitates rapid decision-making, following policies, and not allowing emotions to alter outcomes. However, not every decision is a life-or-death situation, and by analyzing the context and striving to find solutions that benefit the patient and his/her psychological, sociological, and biological circumstances, the provider has a much better opportunity to build a relationship and effectively communicate with both patients and family members.

WHEN CAN MY EMPLOYEE RETURN TO WORK?
31

Before reading the interaction below, please consider the following topics:

Negotiation
- Health communication can be seen as often being a negotiation
- A discussion that includes
  - Problem-solving possibilities
  - Shared understandings
  - Common goals
- Providers and patients are interdependent
  - Patients need providers' knowledge and expertise
  - Providers depend on patients to share information about their problem or situation

Ethics
- To be ethical, providers need to
  - Respect their patients
  - Share information
  - Be honest and truthful
  - Place the good of the patient above the provider's own goals

INITIAL INTERACTION
Role play and/or analyze the following example.
Insert your name and/or profession in the appropriate blanks below.

Frank Carpenter is the owner of a construction firm. One of his employees, John Mayama, was injured on the job two weeks ago, and Mr. Carpenter is calling the provider at the Occupational Medicine Clinic about Mr. Mayama.

Provider:	"Hello. This is ____, and I'm the _____ taking care of Mr. Mayama."
Mr. Carpenter:	"I need to find out what's going on with John; I need him back to work."
Provider:	"He's doing okay, but he's not ready to return to full duty yet."
Mr. Carpenter:	"I know that; he brings me the forms you give him."
Provider:	"Well, under HIPAA, I can't give you any more information."
Mr. Carpenter:	"HIPAA? This is Worker's Compensation. I need to know what's wrong with him and when he'll be back to normal duty."
Provider:	"I can't do that."
Mr. Carpenter:	"Are you new? This is crazy; I pay you all to take care of my employees."
Provider:	"I'll be happy to talk with Mr. Mayama and have him contact you."
Mr. Carpenter:	"You don't have a clue about how this is done!"

Discussion Questions

1. How would you evaluate the communication in this scenario?

   _____

   _____

   _____

   _____

2. Do you agree with the provider that HIPAA laws prevent him/her from discussing the patient's condition with the employer?

   _____

   _____

   _____

   _____

   _____

3. What is the provider's role as it pertains to the employer in this scenario?

_____

_____

_____

_____

4. How do you think the interpersonal communication in this scenario impacts the relationship between the occupational medicine office and the employer?

_____

_____

_____

_____

_____

5. How do government regulations for worker's compensation cases impact the provider–patient relationship? How do they differ from HIPAA regulations?

_____

_____

_____

_____

Interactive Activity

- Rewrite (individually or in a group) the interaction between the provider and the patient's employer.
- Rewrite the conversation, and try to improve the communication effectiveness and information-sharing between the provider and the employer.
- Compare your rewrite to the Alternate Interaction that follows.

Interaction Rewrite

_____

_____

_____

_____

_____

_____

_____

_____

ALTERNATE INTERACTION

Insert your name and/or profession in the appropriate blanks below.

The provider answers the phone.

Provider:	"Hello, Mr. Carpenter. This is _____; I'm a _____."
Mr. Carpenter:	"Hi. I need to find out what's going on with John; I need him back to work."
Provider:	"I understand. John has tendonitis in his shoulder, and is really struggling with his range of motion—he can't raise his arm above his head or reach behind his back."
Mr. Carpenter:	"Okay; but I see him and he doesn't seem to be in much pain."
Provider:	"Well, I think the pain is primarily when he tries to move his shoulder."
Mr. Carpenter:	"So what are we doing to get him well?"
Provider:	"We should have his MRI back this week, and that will confirm if he has torn his rotator cuff or if it's tendonitis."
Mr. Carpenter:	"And then what?"
Provider:	"If it's a torn rotator cuff, he'll need to see an orthopedic surgeon and they'll have to decide if he needs surgery. We've already ordered physical therapy, but we have to wait for the Worker's Compensation insurance to approve it."
Mr. Carpenter:	"So I'm not going to get him back any time soon?"
Provider:	"He can work light duty now; he just can't lift anything with that arm."
Mr. Carpenter:	"That really doesn't help me. We do construction, and there isn't work for one-handed laborers."
Provider:	"Is there something that he could do that would help you, but not require him to lift with that arm?"
Mr. Carpenter:	"I don't know."
Provider:	"Do you have any driving that he could do, and someone else could help him with any lifting?"
Mr. Carpenter:	"Can he drive a stick?"
Provider:	"He probably shouldn't with a bad arm. Do you not have any automatic shift trucks?"
Mr. Carpenter:	"I do—I usually drive it, but I guess I could take one of the standard trucks and let him drive the automatic."
Provider:	"I can okay that, no problem."
Mr. Carpenter:	"Well, that's better I guess, but the automatic has air conditioning."

Provider:	"Sorry, but at least you'll get more use out of John. We should have that MRI report soon and then we'll know more about how long he'll need to be out."
Mr. Carpenter:	"Thanks, that is a big help."
Provider:	"And as soon as we get the MRI results, we'll let John know. So you can make whatever plans are needed."
Mr. Carpenter:	"That would be great. Thanks for trying to make this work better."
Provider:	"No problem; we're trying to help. Be sure to give me a call if you have any more questions."

Follow-up Discussion

1. What are some of the key differences between the two scenarios?

   _____

   _____

   _____

   _____

2. How would you evaluate the provider's handling of this situation?

   _____

   _____

   _____

   _____

3. What specific verbal and nonverbal communication behaviors did the provider use to enhance the interpersonal communication in this scenario?

   _____

   _____

   _____

   _____

4. How did the provider use communication to enhance his/her relationship with the employer?

   _____

   _____

   _____

   _____

5. Do you think negotiating with the employer is ethical? Do you think the patient should be involved in such a discussion?

_____

_____

_____

_____

_____

_____

Key Points

1. Providers must know the rules and regulations related to their roles and the care of their patients. In worker's compensation cases, HIPAA does not apply, and it's not only acceptable to communicate with employers about patients' health, it's required.

2. Worker's compensation and occupational medicine are different co-cultures from traditional provider–patient relationships. In worker's compensation cases, providers must communicate with the patient, the employer, and the Worker's Compensation insurance company. In this co-culture, communication between the provider and the insurance company is even more important than with typical health insurance companies, because no treatment or diagnostic testing can be done without the Worker's Compensation insurance company's approval. In fact, without effective communication between the provider and the Worker's Compensation insurance company, patients may have to wait days, or even weeks, to get diagnostic tests or consultations with specialists. Therefore, providers in this particular setting or co-culture must recognize the differing values and goals from other areas of healthcare. For example, one of the major goals of occupational medicine is to return the patient to work as quickly as is medically warranted. Another unique goal of this co-culture is to meet the employer's expectations in order to maintain their business affiliation. Otherwise, they will send their employees to a different occupational medicine facility. Therefore, negotiation and relationship-building are critically important to caring for the patient, but also to maintaining employers' accounts.

PLEASE TAKE OFF YOUR CLOTHES AND PUT ON THIS GOWN
32

Before reading the interaction below, please consider the following topics:

Intercultural communication
- Providers should avoid ethnocentrism
  - Avoid evaluating patients based on the providers' culture
  - Remain open to the cultural values and beliefs of the patient
- Providers can do a self-assessment to
  - Discover their attitudes toward different cultures
  - Understand their own
    - Communication styles
    - Beliefs
    - Prejudices
- Providers should develop sensitivity to those from different cultures and co-cultures

Ethics
- Avoid intentionally misrepresenting facts or data to manipulate a patient or colleague
- Providers may feel that they know what is best for the patient, but they should avoid disguising information to make it fit their own recommendations
- Require provider honesty in dealings with patients

INITIAL INTERACTION

Role play and/or analyze the following example:

Ahlam is a 30-year-old Arab woman, who is sitting in an examination room with her husband. She is wearing a veil and is fully dressed. This is her first visit to the provider. The provider opens the door, enters the room, and stands near the counter.

Provider:	"Hello."
Mr. Fuhlon:	"My wife is having pain when she goes to the bathroom."
Provider:	"I'd like to talk to her."
Mr. Fuhlon:	"She doesn't speak with men."
Provider:	"Why is that?"
Mr. Fuhlon:	"We are Muslim, and part of our culture is that married women do not talk to men who are not relatives."
Provider:	"I understand, but unfortunately, there's no way for me to confirm that and even if I could, she's an adult and has to give permission for us to talk to anyone."
Mr. Fuhlon:	"She has signed the paper."
Provider:	"I'm really not comfortable with that."
Mr. Fuhlon:	"This is our culture. We have different beliefs from you."
Provider:	"Maybe so, but this is my office, and I can be sued if I don't get a thorough history and do a physical examination."
Mr. Fuhlon:	"You can ask me and I'll tell you. She's never been sick—not in the hospital, nor surgery. She takes no medicines and she has no allergies."
Provider:	"I'm going to need to examine her; will she take off her clothes and put on a gown?"
Mr. Fuhlon:	"Can she leave on her clothes under the gown and you just move them around as you need to?"
Provider:	"I just don't feel comfortable practicing medicine this way, so you'll need to find a different provider."
Mr. Fuhlon:	"Do you not take care of children?"
Provider:	"I do, but it's different."
Mr. Fuhlon:	"I don't think it's different; you let the parents talk for them. I think it's because we are Muslim."

Discussion Questions

1. How would you evaluate the communication in this scenario?

_____

_____

_____

2. How would you assess the cultural issues in this conversation, and how they impact health communication and healthcare delivery?

_____

_____

_____

_____

3. How would you feel as the provider responsible for this patient's care? How would you have handled the situation?

_____

_____

_____

_____

_____

4. What are the ethical issues related to the cultural differences between the provider and the patient's family in this scenario?

_____

_____

_____

_____

5. Discuss how cultural differences between providers and patients can impact health communication, diagnosis, and treatment decisions.

_____

_____

_____

_____

Interactive Activity

- Rewrite (individually or in a group) the interaction between the provider and the patient.
- Rewrite the conversation, and try to improve the communication effectiveness and information-sharing between the provider and the patient or family.
- Compare your rewrite to the Alternate Interaction that follows.

Interaction Rewrite

_____

_____

_____

_____

_____

_____

_____

_____

_____

_____

_____

_____

_____

_____

_____

_____

_____

_____

_____

_____

_____

_____

_____

_____

_____

_____

_____
_____
_____
_____
_____
_____
_____
_____
_____
_____
_____
_____
_____

ALTERNATE INTERACTION

Insert your name and/or profession in the appropriate blanks below.

The provider enters the examination room and walks over to the female patient. The patient's husband steps between the provider and the patient. As they begin to talk, the provider sits down and makes eye contact with the couple.

Provider: "Hello. I'm _____, and I'm a _____."

Mr. Fuhlon: "Hello. My wife is having burning when she goes to the bathroom."

Provider: "Does your wife not speak?"

Mr. Fuhlon: "Our religious beliefs keep her from talking to strangers and from being uncovered around others."

Provider: "I understand and I respect your beliefs. I see she's signed the form saying I can discuss her health with you, so we are okay."

Mr. Fuhlon: "Thank you. Not everyone is so understanding."

Provider:	"I have my own beliefs and I want people to respect them. And with her symptoms, I will likely only need to examine her abdomen, so we can do that without exposing her hardly at all."
Mr. Fuhlon:	"Thank you!"
Provider:	"Because of her complaint and the urine test we did, it seems very likely that she has a urinary tract infection. Has she had many of these?"
Mr. Fuhlon:	"She says no, this is her first."
Provider:	"Okay, and I know she didn't have any fever here, but has she had a temperature above 100 recently?"
Mr. Fuhlon:	"No."
Provider:	"Any abdominal or back pains, or any vomiting?"
Mr. Fuhlon:	"She says no."
Provider:	"Any vaginal bleeding or discharge?"
Mr. Fuhlon:	"Her answer is no."
Provider:	"When we do a urine test, we also do a pregnancy test and that was negative. So here's what is going to happen next. I'm going to examine her and then, if everything is fine, I'll give her a prescription and some instructions."
Mr. Fuhlon:	"Can you stop the burning?"
Provider:	"Yes, one of the medicines should stop it."
Mr. Fuhlon:	"She says thank you and so do I."

Follow-up Discussion

1. How would you compare the two scenarios? What are the key differences?

   _____

   _____

   _____

   _____

2. Do you agree with provider's handling of the situation in the alternate interaction? If so, why? If not, why not?

   _____

   _____

   _____

   _____

3. What did the provider do, verbally and nonverbally, to illustrate her/his respect for the patient's cultural values and beliefs?

_____

_____

_____

_____

4. Do you think the provider's communication and decisions in this example were medically sound? If so, why? If not, why not?

_____

_____

_____

_____

5. How would you compare the ethical issues in these two scenarios?

_____

_____

_____

_____

_____

Key Points

1. Culture plays a critical role in all communication settings. Therefore, providers need to recognize the differences in cultural values and beliefs, and assess how to use communication to build a relationship and accomplish both provider's and patient's goals.
2. Providers constantly determine what information and what physical examination tests they need to assess the patient's complaint. While it may be typical to have a patient undress and put on a gown, there are times when providers can alter their behaviors. Goal attainment in healthcare relies on successful diagnosis and treatment, which in turn requires effective communication. Therefore, providers need to evaluate the intercultural communication, values, beliefs, and goals of patients, and adapt the provider's communication to the patient's needs, whenever possible.
3. Ethical issues abound in healthcare. A provider can say that she/he cannot do a thorough examination if the provider cannot communicate directly with the patient, or have the patient wear a gown. However, if a patient has aphasia or dementia, providers take histories from whomever they can. Therefore, a provider must ask him/herself if it's the patient's cultural beliefs or the patient's requests that are the real issue in such a scenario, and if there are complaints or problems that would require having to expose more of a patient's anatomy. As in this scenario, a provider should be able to work with the patient and her/his family to respect their culture and their needs.

DON'T TELL MY WIFE
SHE'S DYING
33

Before reading the interaction below, please consider the following topics:

End-of-life communication
- In American culture, a difficult topic for most providers, patients, and family members
- To some providers, commitment to health and saving lives makes end-of-life communication seem like giving up
- At some point, will need to be utilized by everyone, either as a patient or a caregiver
- Discussing advanced care directives or living wills with patients is one way to help them handle their final health communication situations

Nonverbal behaviors
- Used to send and receive messages that are not words
- Often trusted more than verbal messages by receivers
- Can be used to reinforce, contradict, or substitute for verbal messages
- Do not have to be intended by the sender to communicate a message to the receiver
- Includes
  - Body Movements
  - Facial expressions
  - Use of space
  - Use of time
  - Touch
  - Clothing and artifacts

INITIAL INTERACTION

Role play and/or analyze the following example:

John Balducci is 72 years old, and he is pacing in his wife, Elizabeth's, hospital room. Elizabeth is 70 years old, and she had a colectomy for colon cancer last year, but was hospitalized two days ago with abdominal pain. The provider enters and Mr. Balducci blocks the path to his wife's bed.

Provider:	"Mr. Balducci?"
Mr. Balducci:	"Can I talk to you—in the hall?"
Provider:	"Okay."
Mr. Balducci:	"Did you get the results back?"
Provider:	"Yes; I was coming to talk with you and Elizabeth."
Mr. Balducci:	"What did the CAT scan show?"
Provider:	"Let's go in so I can talk to both of you about it."
Mr. Balducci:	"I'd rather you tell me first. Please don't tell my wife she's dying."
Provider:	"John, this isn't your decision; she has a right to know."
Mr. Balducci:	"I know my wife—she'll never hear anything except that she's dying, and she won't be able to laugh again."
Provider:	"I'm sorry, but I have an obligation to my patient, so I'm going in there and telling her what we found. Now you can come with me and try to support her, or you can wait out here in the hall; but I'm going in there."
Mr. Balducci:	"Then I want another doctor."
Provider:	"It's not your decision, John. And another doctor will do the same thing."
Mr. Balducci:	"You're going to kill her."
Provider:	"No John, cancer is going to kill her. I'm just going to tell her the truth."

Discussion Questions

1. How would you evaluate the communication in this scenario?

_____

_____

_____

_____

2. What do you think are some of Mr. Balducci's co-cultures that could impact this conversation?

_____

_____

_____

3. If you were the provider, how would you have handled this interaction—in the same way or differently, and why?

_____

_____

_____

_____

4. How do you think the husband's values and beliefs, as compared to the patient's, should be dealt with by the provider?

_____

_____

_____

_____

5. What do you think are the provider's ethical obligations in this scenario?

_____

_____

_____

Interactive Activity

- Rewrite (individually or in a group) the interaction between the provider and the patient's husband.
- Rewrite the conversation, and try to find a way to achieve a more acceptable outcome for the provider, the patient, and Mr. Balducci.
- Compare your rewrite to the Alternate Interaction that follows.

Interaction Rewrite

_____

_____

_____

_____

ALTERNATE INTERACTION

The provider knocks and enters Ms. Balducci's hospital room. Mr. Balducci blocks the path to the bed.

Provider:	"Hi, John."
Mr. Balducci:	"I want to speak with you before you talk to Elizabeth."
Provider:	"Okay, but I'm going to say hello, and then I'll meet you in the hallway."
Mr. Balducci:	"I don't want you talking to her until we talk."
Provider:	"John, I'm happy to talk with you first, but I'm going to say hi to your wife." (The provider walks around Mr. Balducci and over to the bed. The provider touches Ms. Balducci's hand and smiles at her.)
Provider:	"Hi, Elizabeth. How are you doing today?"
Ms. Balducci:	"I'm okay; a little tired. Did you get the report back?"
Provider:	"I did, but John wants to talk to me for just a minute, and then I'll come back and we'll all talk."
Ms. Balducci:	"He doesn't want me to know. He's always trying to protect me."
Provider:	"I understand. I'll be back in just a minute." (The provider goes out into the hall and closes the door to the room.)
Mr. Balducci:	"Don't tell my wife she's dying!" (The provider touches Mr. Balducci on the shoulder.)
Provider:	"John, I know you're worried about how Elizabeth will respond to the news. But I think she's a lot tougher than you think she is."
Mr. Balducci:	"I don't want her to suffer and I don't want her worrying. She worries a lot." (The provider steps in closer to Mr. Balducci, and looking directly into his eyes, speaks more softly than before.)
Provider:	"It sounds like you worry a lot too. Let me ask you this: don't you think Elizabeth would want to know, so she could do some things that she wants to do while she still can? Some people want to travel, some people want to spend more time with their grandchildren, and some folks just want to work in their gardens. But John, she should have the right to decide what she wants to do with whatever time she has left. In some ways she is luckier than other people—some of us don't have that chance, and we never get to put our affairs in order."
Mr. Balducci:	"I don't want to lose her." (He starts to cry and the provider grabs a tissue from a box on the nurse's desk.)

Provider:	"Here John. I completely understand, and remember, no one can predict these things. Let's go inside and talk to Elizabeth together—she's going to do okay with this—and then we can get you all home."
Mr. Balducci:	"I'm scared! What will we do?"
Provider:	"John, I'm going to be here for you both, and we'll talk about some home healthcare to help out."
Mr. Balducci:	"Okay, if we can call you?"
Provider:	"Any time, and she'll be much happier at home."

Follow-up Discussion

1. What are some of the key differences between the two scenarios?

   _____

   _____

   _____

   _____

2. How do you compare the ethical issues in the alternate to the original scenario?

   _____

   _____

   _____

   _____

3. How did the provider in the second scenario enhance the trust and interpersonal relationship with the patient and Mr. Balducci?

   _____

   _____

   _____

   _____

4. How did the provider's nonverbal behaviors impact the outcome of the alternate versus the first scenario?

   _____

   _____

   _____

   _____

Key Points

1. End-of-life communication is difficult enough for providers, but becomes even more challenging when family members make requests that impact the patient's rights and the provider's ethical responsibilities.
2. Interpersonal communication and interpersonal relationships allow providers to communicate with empathy, and to use active listening to provide feedback and support to patients and family members.
3. Nonverbal communication: touch, eye contact, body language, tone of voice, etc., often communicate more than verbal messages. Taking the time to show a patient or a family member that you are listening, and to provide feedback (verbally or nonverbally), can enhance both the communication and the relationship.

INDEX